If you or someone you care for suffers from PMS, this is a book you cannot afford to be without!

PMS:

* why women in their thirties are at highest risk
* why the Pill may trigger PMS
* why PMS may run in families
* why hysterectomies may trigger PMS
* why multiple pregnancies may increase the risk of PMS
* such well-known figures as Mary Todd Lincoln, Joan Crawford, Maria Callas and Queen Victoria may have suffered from PMS
* how lifestyle changes help alleviate PMS symptoms
* the links between PMS and depression, incidents of violence, suicide attempts, alcohol and drug abuse

"Dr. Norris's book is based upon studies conducted with over 2000 women in his clinics, and it includes a program sufferers can use to combat the disorder."
—PITTSBURGH PRESS

PMS

PREMENSTRUAL SYNDROME

Ronald V. Norris, M.D. with Colleen Sullivan

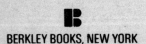

BERKLEY BOOKS, NEW YORK

This Berkley book contains the complete
text of the original hardcover edition.

PMS: PREMENSTRUAL SYNDROME

A Berkley Book / published by arrangement with
Rawson Associates

PRINTING HISTORY
Rawson Associates edition published 1983
Berkley edition / September 1984

ISBN: 0-425-10332-3

A BERKLEY BOOK ® TM 757,375
Berkley Books are published by The Berkley Publishing Group,
200 Madison Avenue, New York, NY 10016.
The name "BERKLEY" and the "B" logo
are trademarks belonging to Berkley Publishing Corporation.

PRINTED IN THE UNITED STATES OF AMERICA

20 19 18 17 16 15 14 13 12 11 10

To / Judy and all the women who suffer from
/ PMS, and to my children: Valerie, Valian,
/ Thane, Lance, Joshua, and angel Sigrid.

Contents

Before You Begin This Book

Contents
(continued)

Acknowledgments

Like most books, this one is the product of the efforts and cooperation of many people. For working so imaginatively and diligently to develop this book, we would like to thank our agent, Susan Cohen.

Orchestrating the many elements of such a wide-ranging project on a very tight deadline was an awesome job, ably undertaken by Lisbeth Bensley, our primary researcher. Alice Weil patiently helped edit the manuscript and added some sorely needed perspective and humor as we struggled toward the finish. To Lis and Alice and a wonderful band of researchers and aides who contributed to the book from London, New York, Boston, and Los Angeles, our gratitude: Barbara Czelusniak, Carole Gould, Eden Graber, Bruce Hager, Sonia Kudla, Sherill Leonard, Valerie and Valian Norris, Robert Rivkin, David Sanger, Stacy Schiff, Fatima Shaik, Kate Stout, Elisa Tinsley, and Christine Ziegler.

This book would not have been possible without the exceptional teachers, mentors, and colleagues who have taught the art and science of medicine and nurtured the belief that the quality of care and the quality of caring are both important in health services: Drs. Arthur Rempel, Fredric Santler, George Ball, at Whitman; Drs. Ray Bunge, Len Heston, Chase Hunter, at Iowa; Drs. David Rogers and Tom Brittingham, at Vanderbilt; Drs. Leon Eisenberg, Seymour Kety, Gerry Klerman, Tom Hackett, and Michael Murphy at Harvard and Massachusetts General Hospital. Drs. Jane Shaw and Peter Ramwell taught the skills and techniques of basic laboratory research at the Worcester Foundation for Experimental Biology. Dr. Charles Lloyd, also of the Worcester Foundation, provided the first introduction to PMS and exposure to clinical research in endocrinology.

Many other physicians, scientists, and other professionals also assisted us by providing material and consenting to interviews. We owe a particular debt to Drs. Willard Allen and William Keye. For their assistance in helping to gather the stories of women coping with PMS, we want to thank Patty Cannon and Lindsey Leckie, co-founders of the National PMS Society, and Virginia Cassara of PMS Action. Most importantly, we owe a very special thanks to the patients evaluated at the Premenstrual Syndrome Program offices and to the hundreds of women with PMS who agreed to be interviewed for this book, freely sharing their experiences and insights so that other women might benefit.

Before You Begin This Book

This book is a celebration of women. It is about women who cope, who have active lives, who juggle responsibilities of work and home, who raise children, who run businesses, who are warm and loving mates cherished by their families and friends. It is also a book about pain, a cyclical kind of physical and psychological pain that intrudes into the lives and consciousness of millions of women around the globe. Five to ten percent of all women — nearly seven million Americans and more than one hundred million women worldwide — find themselves struggling every month, for a few days or as long as three weeks, to deal with a menstrually-related illness known as premenstrual syndrome, or PMS. This book is for these women, their families, and friends.

We first became aware of the existence of premenstrual syndrome about fourteen years ago while completing a fellowship with Dr. Charles Lloyd, a well-known reproductive endocrinologist, at the Worcester Foundation for Experimental Biology in Massachusetts, where the birth control pill was initially developed. A number of women seen in the Endocrine Clinic of the foundation suffered from PMS. Further, while carrying out a study of aggression in women, we found that six women imprisoned for murder all had committed the murders the day before or the first day of their menstrual period. The connection seemed too solid to be mere coincidence. In subsequent years we also saw the symptoms of premenstrual syndrome in women we knew personally, in some women with whom we worked, as well as in patients we were treating for other problems. We diagnosed the conditions as best we could at the time and treated them with varying degrees of success. It was only after my wife developed PMS and I became aware of its deleterious impact upon her, our relationship, and our family that I recognized the significance of the disorder. I began to study the statistics and scientific literature, and came to appreciate how little understanding American women and their physicians had of this disorder. Our interest in the syndrome resulted in a decision to open the first center in the United States specializing in PMS diagnosis and treatment in 1981 and to establish a foundation to foster research in and education about PMS and similar disorders. Since 1981, more than two thousand women have been evaluated for the condition at our centers.

Based on the findings from our practice, we developed this book. Its purpose is not only to educate and inform the public about premenstrual syndrome as a treatable medical condition, but also to describe the wide-ranging impact of PMS on the home, family, and friends, in the workplace and in social situations. We've also examined the profound legal and social implications of the condition — our rebuttal to the debate that has developed over PMS as a legal defense and as a possible obstacle to the equal rights movement for women.

With the cooperation and assistance of many of our patients, we have gathered the stories of those who know what it's like to live with PMS. We asked the women we interviewed to speak freely about their experiences and the effect the disorder has had on their personal and professional lives and relationships — and they did. Unfortunately, most women feel that a stigma attaches to the PMS condition; they're probably right. We hope that as information about PMS and its treatment becomes available, PMS will be no more onerous a burden than the common cold. Today, however, most women do not want to be identified as suffering from the syndrome. Thus to preserve their privacy, we have changed the names and in many cases the occupations and geographic locations of the women we interviewed.

The identities of physicians and other experts cited throughout the book have not been changed, however.

For those readers who think they may have premenstrual syndrome, we suggest that you read this book carefully, especially Section VI on diagnosis and lifestyle changes. But we urge you to consult your own physician before undertaking a self-diagnosis. While too few physicians evaluate and treat PMS in this country now, the growing demand for such care will undoubtedly result in more and more physicians recognizing and treating the syndrome in the months and years to come. By reading this book and becoming informed health-care consumers, women can help their physicians become educated about PMS, too. And that's a first step toward improving medical care for PMS sufferers.

SECTION I / *The Basics*

Chapter 1

*"But it's always interesting when one doesn't
see. If you don't see what a thing means,
you must be looking at it wrong way round."*

Agatha Christie

PMS: What It Is and What It Isn't

Premenstrual syndrome, or PMS, is a defect of physiology, not of character. In extreme cases, its effects are so far-reaching that it may become difficult to separate the syndrome from the personality. Most women, perhaps eighty-five percent of the menstruating female population, have experienced symptoms of PMS in the days preceding their menstrual period, even if for some it might involve just one cycle out of twenty. About forty percent of all menstruating women — nearly twenty-seven million Americans — experience fairly regular symptoms of premenstrual syndrome. For the vast majority, PMS occurs as mild complaints — including irritability, bloating, and headaches — simply signalling that the menstrual flow will start within hours or days. It is a minor, if recurring, inconvenience. Five to ten percent of menstruating women, however, suffer from severe PMS. For these women — three million to seven million Americans — the days prior to the onset of menstruation are marked by a gamut of physiological and psychological symptoms that disrupt their personal and professional lives.

PMS is a complex disorder apparently linked to the cyclic activity of the hypothalamic-pituitary-ovarian axis. It is associated with a wide range of symptoms recurring regularly at the same phase of each menstrual cycle followed by a symptom-free phase in each cycle. The symptoms include irritability, tension, headache, depression, fatigue, breast swelling and tenderness, abdominal bloating, weight gain, increased thirst or appetite, cravings for sweet or salty foods, acne, asthma, and constipation. Other symptoms that may occur on a regular, cyclical basis include:

- *Boils, herpes, hives*
- *Epilepsy, migraines, dizziness*
- *Conjunctivitis, sties, uveitis*
- *Hoarseness, sore throat, sinusitis, rhinitis*
- *Cystitis, urethritis*
- *Child abuse, alcohol abuse, assaults, panic attacks, psychotic episodes, suicide attempts*

To women with PMS, confronted each month by the same pains, depression or feelings of being out of control, Edna St. Vincent Millay's aphorism is particularly apt: "It's not true that life is one damn thing after another — it's one damn thing over and over." For women with mild conditions, her flippancy is on target; but those with very severe cases endure an anguish and agony that more accurately parallel that of Hamlet's father's ghost:

> "Doomed for a certain term to walk the night,
> And for the day confined to fast in fires."

The PMS disorder was first described in a scientific paper published in 1931 by Dr. Robert Frank. Today medical textbooks ignore or barely mention the syndrome and its multiplicity of symptoms. As a result, most physicians — male doctors who haven't studied PMS in medical school and never experienced a menstrual cycle — either dismiss it as a psychosomatic phenomenon or misdiagnose it. Yet, quite clearly, the condition exists. Despite the prevailing attitude, more than one hundred research studies on premenstrual syndrome and cyclic disorders related to menstruation have been published over the years. More painfully, it has damaged millions of lives, and contributed to divorce, child abuse, alcoholism, and violence, hamstrung careers, and hindered personal development.

Why does the medical establishment keep the blinders on? Despite the recent and rapid increase in the number of women practicing medicine, the prevalent view of the female body remains male-oriented, in the male-dominated medical and psychiatric establishments. As Paula Weideger writes in *Menstruation and Menopause*, "Gynecology textbooks are riddled with statements about the psychological or sociological roots of menstrual and menopausal distress. Despite feelings of vulnerability and menstrual shame, women have repeatedly attempted to tell their physicians that the problems are not in their heads but in their bodies. The doctor, convinced his theory is the right one, pays little attention to what his patient has to say.''

To many gynecologists, pain is the most decisive evidence that a woman has failed to accept the female role. This has led to a vicious circle in which women suffer the most severe discomfort, go to a doctor for help, are told they are psychologically responsible for their pain, and leave the doctor's office in physical and mental agony.

Thousands, if not hundreds of thousands, of laypeople — especially the relatives, spouses and children of women who suffer from PMS, if not the women themselves — long ago linked certain recurring behavior and physical complaints to the menstrual cycle. It is such a common problem, in fact, that it has entered our popular literature, almost without notice or comment. Two authors of novels published in this country have woven their plots around the lives of women with severe PMS: *The Third Deadly Sin* by Lawrence Sanders, the best-selling murder mystery, and *I Am Mary Dunne,* a psychological study of insanity, by Canadian writer Brian Moore. It must be emphasized that the central characters of these works are tormented by the most extreme type of PMS, the depths of which only a very small percentage of women are likely to know. Both authors developed their characters because they had known women who suffered from the premenstrual syndrome. Lawrence Sanders researched PMS and the host of physical and psychological disorders of his protaganist for two years before writing his book. Brian Moore says he was in love with a woman who had PMS. "For two weeks she was normal. But her personality changed very rapidly, to the day,'' he told us in an interview. "If we ever had any dinner engagements during this time, we could never go. And it interfered with her work. She was a highly trained, highly educated woman who had a very responsible job. However, when the symptoms developed, she had to be out of the office. Consequently, she had to work nights during her normal time to compensate.''

The memories of that troubled existence led him to shape his character Mary Dunne in his friend's image. "Almost every woman I know has some personality change" (due to her menstrual cycle). "We can't dismiss it. Premenstrual tension differs greatly (from one person to another) and women who suffer from it badly see it affect their jobs, their relationships, their lives.''

The Menstrual Cycle

To understand PMS, you first have to understand the most delicate and sophisticated function of the female body, the menstrual cycle.

The control center of a number of body systems, including the sex hormones, is the hypothalamus. Each month from menarche on, this walnut-sized unit buried deeply in the brain acts as elegant interpreter of the body's rhythms, transmitting messages to the pituitary gland that set the menstrual cycle in motion. The pituitary, in turn, responds by producing two critical hormones: the Follicle Stimulating Hormone, known as FSH, and the Luteinizing Hormone, or LH. From first menstrual cycle to menopause, the hypothalamus acts as the conductor of a highly trained orchestra. Once its baton signals the downbeat to the pituitary, the hypothalamus-pituitary-ovarian axis is united in purpose and begins to play its symphonic message, preparing a woman's body for conception and child-bearing.

There are two phases to the monthly cycle, identified by the dominance of the hormone during each part: the follicular phase and the luteal phase.

In the follicular phase, FSH is secreted into the bloodstream and reaches the ovary, where it does just what its name promises: it stimulates the development of the follicles of the ovary that contain egg cells. (Usually only one ovary and fifteen to twenty follicles are stimulated in a single cycle.) At the same time, the endometrium, or uterine lining, starts to develop and thicken in preparation for the potential implantation of a fertilized egg. The follicles start to develop, vying against each other for a dominant role, like violinists competing for the position of concertmaster. After the fifth day, a dominant follicle emerges, fated to grow into an egg. The others wither and die off, while FSH secretion stimulates the remaining follicle to manufacture estrogen, another sex hormone. On the 11th and 12th days, a burst of estrogen is emitted from the follicle like a clap of tympani; this is the signal to the pituitary that the follicle is about to produce an egg. The pituitary responds with an answering explosion of LH, which lasts for two or three days, overriding the influence of FSH and jolting the ovary into producing an egg. Within thirty-six hours the crescendo is heard: the ovary erupts with the egg.

Ovulation marks the beginning of the fourteen-day luteal phase. (The length of a menstrual cycle varies, but the luteal phase lasts fourteen days. In the textbook example of a twenty-eight-day cycle, the follicular and luteal phases are both fourteen days. In a forty-day cycle, the luteal phase is fourteen days and the follicular phase is twenty-six days. Ovulation would occur on the last day of the follicular phase or the twenty-sixth day, not at the midpoint, or the twentieth day.) The egg leaves the ovary, passing through the Fallopian tubes to the uterus, where it may or may not be fertilized by male sperm. The follicle, now empty, changes character in response to the secretion of LH and becomes the corpus luteum, or yellow body. The corpus luteum manufactures and secretes progesterone and estrogens. The subsequent high concentration of estrogen in the bloodstream and pituitary inhibits the secretion of any more FSH or LH, which prevents them from signalling the ovary to develop any new follicles during this cycle.

If the egg that has been released is fertilized and a fetus conceived in the cycle, the corpus luteum flourishes. Enormous amounts of progesterone will be secreted to nurture and sustain the development of the fetus until the placenta takes over. Most cycles, however, do not result in pregnancy. In these cycles, then, the production of progesterone continues until a critical level is reached. When the pituitary detects that enough progesterone is in the bloodstream, it slows the production of LH. As LH production declines, the corpus luteum is no longer being fueled and it begins to decay. As the corpus luteum wanes, the amount of progesterone and estrogen being produced decreases. When the production of progesterone and estrogen reach their nadirs, menstruation begins. The uterus is no longer stimulated by the hormones and the endometrium — the lining of the uterus — begins to slough off. After the first day or two of flow, the pituitary responds to the absence of estrogen and progesterone by making more FSH and preparing for the next cycle.

In some women, however, the delicate multi-system effort of the menstrual cycle is thrown out of balance. The result: not a symphonic serenade, but an atonal cacophony. In some women, an imbalance in one or many elements of the hypothalamic-pituitary-ovarian axis produces the premenstrual syndrome: a Rabelaisian nightmare, a dissonance "above the pitch, out of tune, and off the hinges."

Reproductive Hormones

The sex hormones, estrogen, progesterone and the androgens (of which testosterone is the dominant substance), are all derived from cholesterol; they serve as blood-borne messengers from the glands that secrete them to the target organs that utilize them. Hormones act upon their specific target organ by quickening the rate of internal cellular reactions. Estrogen and progesterone are believed to act as gene activators. Once inside the nucleus of the cell, the hormone activates the gene, initiating the synthesis of protein, and eventually influences all of the characteristic functions of that cell.

Estrogen is present in both males and females, secreted by the adrenal gland. In the female body it stimulates the development of breasts and the reproductive organs. It is also responsible for feminine curves, the fatty deposits necessary to support reproduction. It acts on both sexes in fat metabolism and the production of blood proteins as well as vascular and muscle tissue. Estrogen's primary function is in the menstrual cycle and the maintenance of the fetus. During the cycle, as follicles ripen in the ovary under the influence of FSH, they begin to secrete estrogen. The hormone travels back to the pituitary, and there activates the surge in LH which leads to ovulation. After ovulation the corpus luteum continues the follicle's job of producing estrogen, as well as progesterone. To facilitate the sperms' journey to the egg, estrogen also increases and thins out the cervical mucus, giving the sperm easier access to the uterus. And estrogen assists the egg's journey to the uterus by increasing the motility of the Fallopian tubes. The hormone further contributes to the reproductive process by nurturing the growth of the uterine endometrium that will eventually anchor and feed the fertilized egg.

In concert with its male analog, testosterone, estrogen halts bone development during adolescence by sealing the cartilage ends of the bones. A deficiency in estrogen leads to osteoporosis, a common disorder in post-menopausal women. Estrogen also accelerates the synthesis of the blood proteins and the metabolism of fatty acids which inhibits the production of cholesterol. It appears to protect women from heart disease and arteriosclerosis; women's incident rates of heart disease are much lower than men's but do increase in post-menopausal women. And estrogen also stimulates gland secretions in the skin and plays a role in normal vascular maintenance; estrogen deficiency, such as that experienced at menopause, is marked by hot flashes.

Progesterone helps ready the endometrium for the implantation of a fertilized egg and sustains the fetus during pregnancy. Progesterone is estrogen-dependent; it requires prior stimulation by estrogen to do its work. Estrogen initially stimulates the growth of the endometrium, then progesterone steps in to convert the tissue into active glands. Under the influence of progesterone, the glands fill with glycogen to feed the fetus, blood vessels proliferate, and enzymes accumulate, ready to aid in the fetus' growth. Like estrogen, progesterone is initially secreted by the ovary's corpus luteum, later by the placenta. One of its functions is to prevent another egg from being fertilized once one is in place in the uterus. After fertilization, it causes the cervical mucus to become thick and sticky, which locks sperm out and further protects the fertilized egg and uterus from bacteria. Progesterone also elevates the body temperature slightly, which is why we can determine the time of ovulation and peak fertility by tracking a woman's temperature.

In men, the principal sex hormone is testosterone, secreted by the testes. It is responsible for the production of sperm, the development and maintenance of male reproductive organs and secondary sex characteristics such as pubic hair, the deepened voice, coarser skin texture, thicker secretion of oil by the skin glands, and male muscle and fat distribution. It accounts for sex drive and growth — in both men and women; the adrenal glands produce small amounts of testosterone in women. This hormone also accounts for the greater aggressiveness of males.

Physical, emotional, and behavioral changes can be tied to the cyclical pattern of sex hormone activity and to the changes of hormone supply between one cycle of life and the next. The pattern of hormone production is different for males and females; this contributes to sexual differences in physical and emotional experience, as well as differences in behavior. While females have a distinct, observable cycle that makes changes in their behavior or temperament easy to mark in terms of the cycle, males also exhibit recurring patterns of behavior that some researchers believe correspond to a cycling of hormonal levels. In men, however, these shifts are often attributed to "moodiness." The ebb and flow of male hormones are not as dramatic as those in women but they are observable. In some men a stretch of good-neutral-bad temper occurs at regular intervals — thirty days, forty days, fifty-five days, or so on — that is observed by family, friends, and co-workers who adapt their own behavior toward and expectations of the men to account for the mood swings.

A 1970 study, reporting on sixteen years of data collected by Danish researchers, showed that men experience a definite thirty-day cycle of testosterone production. A 1969 study undertaken by the Omi Railway Company of Japan reported that male workers had predictable cycles that affected their work efficiency, decision-making, and proneness to accidents. The railroad revised its work schedules to remove employees from critical duties during their "bad" or unpredictable phases. Dr. Franz Halberg of the University of Minnesota is continuing his research into cyclical behavior in males; to date he has found evidence of cyclical surges and declines in grip strength and beard growth due to changes in hormonal levels. As Dr. Estelle Ramey, a professor of physiology at the Georgetown University School of Medicine, has observed, "In healthy maturity, the adult human changes with clocklike regularity during each day, just as he or she does during each month, or each life's season." If the hormonal shifts in males were as sharp as those in women and contributed to as many medical problems, one could be certain that the validity of the condition would not be in question.

Eleven Landmarks

Premenstrual syndrome can be difficult to identify and diagnose because its symptoms encompass so many systems of the body. With PMS, one size simply does not fit all. The landmarks of PMS that can aid women and their physicians in identifying the condition are:

• *Time of onset.* PMS tends to begin at puberty, after pregnancy, after termination of the birth control pill, or after an episode of amenorrhea (no periods).

• *Time of increased severity.* Mild symptoms of PMS may be present for a number of years but the woman notes a marked increase in her symptoms following the discontinuance of the birth control pill, following a pregnancy, after the cessation of breastfeeding, after a tubal ligation or hysterectomy, or after an episode of amenorrhea.

• *Painless menstruation*. Although pelvic discomfort or pain may occasionally be a part of the premenstrual syndrome, painful menstruation is not.

• *Weight fluctuations*. Many women with PMS experience monthly weight swings of six to nine pounds, and over the years experience weight ranges of twenty-eight pounds or more. The proper comparison is made between the highest-ever weight, excluding pregnancy, with the lowest-ever weight by history.

• *Food cravings*. Hunger and eating binges, especially involving sweet or salty foods, are often noted in the premenstruum. The onset of acute symptoms, violent episodes, panic attacks, and migraine headaches often occur after an absence of food intake exceeding four or five hours.

• *Intolerance for alcohol*. Women suffering from PMS may notice a decreased tolerance for alcohol during the premenstruum, accompanied by alcohol cravings.

• *Inability to tolerate the birth control pill*. Women with premenstrual syndrome often experience weight gain, depression, headaches, and exacerbation of the premenstrual syndrome symptoms with the use of birth control pills.

• *History of postpartum depression*. The depression must have been of sufficient severity to require psychiatric treatment or admission to a hospital. A study of one hundred women admitted to the hospital for severe premenstrual syndrome revealed that seventy-three percent of those who had been pregnant had suffered from significant postpartum depression.

• *History of threatened abortion*. Bleeding in the early months of pregnancy followed by a successful pregnancy is relatively common in PMS cases.

• *History of hypertension or toxemia during pregnancy*. Studies show that eighty-six percent of women who have had a pregnancy complicated by toxemia subsequently developed premenstrual syndrome.

• *Increased sex drive*. Women suffering from PMS may experience an increase in libido during the premenstrual phase. By contrast, women suffering from PMS as well as depression may experience a decreased interest in sex.

Timing is Critical

The key to the diagnosis of PMS is not so much the identifying of signs or symptoms as it is establishing the timing of the symptoms in relation to the menstrual cycle. Several typical patterns are symptoms that begin:

- *One to ten days prior* to menstruation and continue until the onset of menstruation.
- *At ovulation*, resolve in a day or two, and then reappear later in the premenstrual phase.
- *At ovulation*, continuing until the onset of menstruation.
- *At ovulation*, continue steadily into the menstrual period, resolving only toward the end of the menstrual period. These women often complain that they only have one good week per month.

Each pattern must be followed by a symptom-free phase lasting at least seven days to constitute a diagnosis of PMS.

Signs of other chronic disorders, including depression, rheumatoid arthritis, ulcerative colitis, and asthma may be present throughout the month in varying degrees, but worsen in the days before menstrual flow. Such instances do NOT represent the premenstrual syndrome. But it is possible for a woman to have one of these conditions, in addition to others, AND premenstrual syndrome concurrently. This is not unusual in the more severe cases.

Other Menstrually-Related Disorders

Premenstrual syndrome is commonly misdiagnosed. Among the conditions it has been mistaken for are:

Dysmenorrhea — pelvic pain or menstrual cramping, generally beginning one day prior to the onset of menstruation and ending during or with the end of the flow.

Endometriosis — a painful condition marked by severe cramps and heavy bleeding that results when endometrial tissue (the lining of the uterus) appears and proliferates outside of the uterus, clinging to the ovaries, uterine ligaments, vagina, vulva, cervix, intestines, or pelvic lymph glands. In rare cases endometriosis may spread to the kidney, lungs, arms, hands, thighs, or spleen.

Pelvic Inflammatory Disease — an umbrella term for various types of infections of the uterus, Fallopian tubes, ovaries and adjacent tissues, marked by severe pelvic and abdominal pain or abdominal swelling, nausea, vomiting, and high fever.

Some psychological conditions are also confused with PMS. Among them are:

Cyclothymic Disorder — a condition characterized by numerous periods of depression and other symptoms over a period of at least two years, but not severe enough to meet the criteria of a major depressive episode.

Dysthymic Disorder — depressive neurosis, characterized by a chronic mood disturbance of about two year's duration and a loss of interest in most activities. Symptoms include social withdrawal, tearfulness, extreme pessimism, and decreased functioning at work, home, or school.

Major Depressive Episode — condition marked by loss of interest or pleasure in all activities. Symptoms are persistent depression, hopelessness, sadness, and/or irritability.

What Causes PMS?

Why do some women have severe premenstrual syndrome and others no symptoms at all? Why do some women have mild cases while others make the rounds of doctors' offices seeking help? As Dr. William Keye, a reproductive endocrinologist and assistant professor of obstetrics and gynecology at the University of Utah Medical Center, says, "The real problem is, we don't know."

We don't know, but we have suspicions. Many theories have been proposed as to the cause of premenstrual syndrome. The most frequently discussed is that advanced by Dr. Katharina Dalton, the British pioneer in the field, who suggests that a deficiency of progesterone in relation to the amount of estrogen present before menstruation triggers the syndrome. Others suggest that perhaps the ovaries in some women produce a substance that sets off a reaction or imbalance in the endocrine system, or that an aberrant estrogen is at the bottom of it all. We think it is much more complicated than that. First of all, premenstrual syndrome is now a catchall phrase encompassing more than one hundred fifty symptoms that occur cyclically in some women. That is a very strong indication that we are not talking about one syndrome, but several. They may be the red flags of several different malfunctions of the endocrine system; or they could result from a central malfunction that affects many systems of the body, producing different reactions — or symptoms — from more than one system.

We also know that the tools of scientific research make it possible to identify the causes of PMS if the proper questions are posed, if sufficient money is made available to support the studies, and if the research is undertaken by top medical investigators on a systematic basis. Research into PMS is not nearly as problematic as trying to find a cure for cancer. And while the research is being done, we know — from clinical experience — that PMS can be treated and eliminated. Women no longer have to suffer in silence. With proper screening procedures, an accurate diagnosis of PMS can be made, and the condition treated with a combination of lifestyle changes and, if necessary, progesterone.

Facing Up to PMS

Many women suffering from PMS have visited and been examined by more than one physician — usually three and sometimes as many as twenty specialists, including gynecologists, internists, psychiatrists, endocrinologists, neurologists, and neurosurgeons. Their dilemma is that expressed by Alexander Pope in his *Moral Essays:* "Who shall decide when doctors disagree?" Because the medical profession, outside of a handful of physicians, has failed to recognize that pain and problems do accompany the menstrual cycle, enormous numbers of women are suffering. They are not fantasizing or imagining their symptoms. Most women have been ignored, misdiagnosed, or mistreated for their condition.

Is it any wonder then that women are the dominant health care consumers in this country? Sixty percent of all patient visits to physicians are made by women. The difference in health-care-seeking behavior between men and women starts at puberty, studies show. Boys and girls see physicians roughly with the same degree of frequency. Younger males, in fact, take a slight lead in the number of visits. But after puberty, the picture shifts dramatically. There is a sharp increase on the part of females, and a decrease in the number of visits by males. This pattern will persist throughout adulthood.

A variety of medications have been tried in PMS cases. But most women report that the typical medications make their symptoms worse, have no effect at all, result in significant side effects, alleviate some of their symptoms, but not all, or work for a few months and then no longer help. Among the medications that do not appear to resolve PMS are: diuretics, oral contraceptives, tranquilizers, antidepressants, lithium, bromocriptine, prostaglandin inhibitors, and vitamin therapy.

To overcome the damage that this lack of proper diagnosis and treatment has caused, education is sorely needed. If you're one of the millions of women confronted by a confusing array of physical and psychological events each month, you need information about the condition and reassurance that the problems are part of a biological condition. It has a name; it is not psychosomatic; it is not your imagination playing tricks on you; you are not losing your grip on sanity; you are not lacking in discipline or will to overcome it. For many, just being told that the pain is real helps to allay the fears, the despair, and the blow to self-esteem.

Changes in lifestyle and other therapy may be necessary to treat PMS. Reduction of stress, exercise, and careful attention to diet and nutrition can all help. Some women with mild or moderate cases of PMS find that the lifestyle changes alone resolve their problems. For the most severe cases, though, these help but do not eliminate the PMS symptoms. For these cases, we use progesterone, a therapy that long clinical use has demonstrated to be the most effective treatment. Progesterone seems to alleviate the greatest number of symptoms with the fewest side effects of any of the medications used to treat the disorder.

Chapter 2

> *"Nothing could easily be found that is more*
> *remarkable than the monthly flux of women.*
> *Contact with it turns new wine sour, crops*
> *touched by it become barren, grafts die,*
> *seeds in gardens are dried up, the fruit of*
> *trees fall off, the bright surface of mirrors*
> *in which it is merely reflected is dimmed, the*
> *edge of steel and gleam of ivory are dulled,*
> *hives of bees die, even bronze and iron are at*
> *once seized by rust, and a horrible smell fills*
> *the air: to taste it drives dogs mad and effects*
> *their bite with an incurable poison."*
>
> Pliny the Elder, **Natural History**

Eve's Curse

Primitive societies associated menstruation with ill fortune, disasters, and the supernatural. Aristotle asserted that the "glance of a menstrual woman takes the polish from a mirror and the person who next glances in it will be bewitched." Pliny indicated that uncovering the body of a woman during her menstrual flow empowered her to stop hailstorms, whirlwinds, and lightning. During her menstrual flow, a woman was in contact with the stars and capable of magic, Aelion believed. This connection of menstruation with the supernatural seemed logical enough to early cultures: how else did women continue to thrive each month after suffering inexplicable and recurring bleeding, bleeding that did not result in death or stem from bodily injury? Like the phoenix arising from the ashes, women were clearly special, endowed with powers unknown to mere males. But the males were in control, after all. Instead of according women special status and honors for their rejuvenative feats, the men scrutinized this monthly phenomena and concluded that it was accompanied by strange and sometimes unacceptable behavior. From Hippocrates on, healers cited mental disturbances arising from the association of guilt and fear with menstruation. Women were flawed, not blessed, with this cycle of blood.

Some societies ensured a safe distance between menstruating women and others by banishing the women during their flow to special areas — tents, huts, a hillside — set aside for this purpose. This taboo was enforced to protect the group from damage to the crops and from the outbursts or behavior that were associated with menstruating women. Some of these cultures apparently thought there was a poison or "menotoxin" in the menstrual blood. In part, this idea was inferred from the dramatic changes in bodily functions, attitude, and behavior that some evinced each month just prior to the menstrual flow. As soon as the flow began, or within a few days of it, the women's behavior would return to a normal state. To primitive peoples, then, it was assumed that a toxic agent or spirit had caused the dramatic changes prior to menstruation and that once the menstrual flow began the toxin was eliminated or washed away in the menstrual blood.

Freud and others rejected these theories about menstrual taboos on various grounds. Freud felt the theory of man's fear and horror of blood was exaggerated since it did not suppress customs such as circumcision of boys or the cruel extirpation of the clitoris and labia minora of girls, a practice which continues in some parts of the Middle East and Africa even today. Instead, these critics created a view of their own, a view to which few, if any, women we've ever met subscribe. Freudian theory suggested that women's envy and desire for the male sex organ and their anger and frustration at not having one led them to act out, emotionally or with otherwise inexplicable episodes of "hysteria," temporary paralysis, and a gamut of psychosomatic diseases. The males, in turn, sought to distance themselves and the community from these episodes, which fostered the creation of taboos. This theory undoubtedly reinforced Freud's self-satisfaction but it has very little to do with how women today — and probably in the past — perceived themselves and their sexuality.

As Sheila MacLeod so eloquently stated in *The Art of Starvation*, describing her experience at menarche: "I'm sorry to disappoint orthodox Freudians, but I felt no penis envy, and I didn't think myself to be maimed in any way... I was horrified and disgusted by menstruation rather than by sexuality. I felt that some dreadful punishment had been visited upon me, punishment for a crime which I had never committed. But I think I knew unconsciously that the supposed crime was twofold: I was being punished for being female and for having grown up." As she noted, this sense of punishment is felt by girls, not boys, in adolescence because the physical changes of girls traditionally were not considered an appropriate topic for open discussion. The development of boys, on the other hand, was and is treated as a mark of manhood.

Despite the advances in science and education over time, the superstitions and peculiar notions surrounding menstruation stubbornly persisted into the 19th Century. As late as 1878 the *British Medical Journal* published lengthy, earnest correspondence as to whether a menstruating woman would contaminate the food she touches. One writer, opposed to medical education for women, exclaimed: "If such bad results accrue curing dead meat while she is menstruating, what would result, under similar conditions, from her attempt to cure living flesh in her midwifery or surgical practice?"

S. Icard, a noted French physician, writing in 1890, stated that "the psychical and physical state of women during the menstrual periods seems to me to constitute one of the chief reasons why she should not administer public affairs. Indeed, one cannot depend upon a health so fragile and so often disturbed; the errs of judgments and false evaluations so often made at that time prove that they [women] are unable to undertake comfortably and successfully that which should be the exclusive lot of the strong sex."

To these sexist opinions came a slew of women's voices shooting down the specious theories. Dr. Mary Jacobi presented a rigorous defense in her book, *The Question of Rest for Women During Menstruation,* published in 1876. In 1914, Leta Hollingworth, in her book *Functional Periodicity: An Experimental Study of the Mental and Motor Abilities of Women During Menstruation,* noted that "the tradition emanating from the mystic and romantic novelists, that woman is a mysterious being, half hysteric, half angel, has found its way into scientific writing. Through the centuries gone, those who wrote were men, and since the phenomenon of periodicity was foreign to them, they not unnaturally seized upon it as a probable source of the alleged 'mystery' and 'caprice' of womankind. The dogma once formulated has been quoted on authority from author to author until the present day. A more immediate source of error is to be noted in the fact that the greater part of the evidence quoted on this subject is clinical in character, the contribution of physicians [male]. But it should be obvious to the least critical mind that normal women do not come under the care and observation of physicians.''

Hollingworth went for the jugular in challenging the basis of the male argument: ''Men to whom it would never have occurred to write authoritatively on any other subject regarding which they possessed no reliable or expert knowledge, have not hesitated to make the most positive statements regarding the mental and motor abilities of women as related to functional periodicity… It is positively asserted that women cannot successfully pursue professional and industrial life because they are incapacitated, and should rest for one-fifth of their time; yet it is not proposed that mothers, housekeepers, cooks, scrub women, and dancers should be relieved periodically from their labors and responsibilities.''

From the dawn of time until well into the 20th Century women have had to defend themselves against male attacks on their abilities, despite the myriad responsibilities and skills they juggled effortlessly day after day, generation to generation. Man's fears and awe of woman, especially of her generative powers, have probably played some part in the reluctance of society in general —and the male-dominated medical profession in particular — to recognize and deal with premenstrual syndrome.

Uncovering the Medical Evidence

We know, of course, how the feminist debate has turned out — up to a point. Women have seized an equal role in all aspects of society, proving that they can fight fires, graduate from West Point, win election to political office, or become lawyers, physicians, accountants, truck drivers, ministers, and rabbis — and still be wives and mothers, should they choose to do so. All things are not equal though: while more than half of all adult women are in the workforce, they earn on average fifty-nine cents for every one dollar a man makes. But all in all, women's progress has been rapid, forceful, and successful in almost every facet of life in this country. Every facet but one. Women's medical problems have always gotten short shrift in this country. A belated acknowledgment of this was made in 1982 with the release of a scientific study noting that women's pain and discomfort, especially during the morning sickness of pregnancy and at menstruation, has been significantly underestimated and downplayed by physicians. Since more than four hundred thousand physicians in this country are male and about sixty thousand are female, the underestimation could well be due to the fact that a man has never experienced the reproductive incidents that a woman goes through and cannot comprehend the extent of the trauma.

The shortsightedness is apparent in the medical profession's attitude toward premenstrual syndrome. A review of the medical literature reveals that a lot of doctors have seen PMS in their practices, some have treated it, some have written about it, and hundreds of thousands of practitioners have read about it in clinical journals. But that's where it was left until recently. Why? Well, it is a woman's complaint, after all. And, as Food and Drug Administration officials pointed out a few years ago, it isn't life-threatening. To some physicians, then, premenstrual syndrome is not a priority. Many doctors view any discomfort arising from menstruation as normal, simply part of the woman's burden. To be fair, we must emphasize that because the symptoms of PMS cut across so many systems of the body and thus so many medical specialties, many cases of PMS are not properly diagnosed because no single physician has observed or been told of the spectrum of symptoms the patient has. The emphasis on specialization in modern medicine thus contributes to the confusion over and lack of recognition of PMS.

There is a trove of scientific evidence and published papers citing the existence of a battery of health problems and behavioral changes in women prior to the onset of menstruation. The first paper to do so in this country dates back more than fifty years. The first paper to do so worldwide was published in 1842, more than one hundred forty years ago. A prominent endocrinologist, Dr. Robert T. Frank of New York, is credited with first describing the scope of the syndrome in a paper published in 1931, *"The Hormonal Causes of Premenstrual Tension."* In his book published in 1929, *The Female Sex Hormone*, he described the recurring premenstrual problems of breast swelling and tenderness, headaches, edema of the eyelids, cheeks and extremities, hives, herpes simplex, abdominal discomfort, and "uncontrollable irritation and depression which manifests itself in manic or melancholic crises." He also noted that the number of suicides among women was highest during the time immediately prior to menstruation.

Other scientists had connected the onset of menstruation with health complaints even before Frank published his works. A monograph by Brierrede Boismont was published in Paris in 1842 concerning the relationship of menstruation and the mental state. He noted that various "low grade psychotic tendencies" appeared at this time. Other researchers published clinical papers noting a relationship between menstruation and genital herpes, periodic jaundice, gall bladder attacks, skin disorders, metabolic changes, a range of ophthalmological disorders including conjunctivitis, scleritis, iritis, herpes, corneae, and retinitis, even detachment of the retina. From 1900 until the publication of Frank's work in 1931, more than twenty papers appeared in clinical publications linking regular, periodic occurrence of various disorders during the premenstrual phase. Among them: arthritis, epilepsy, edema, skin disorders, headaches, and psychoses.

Frank opened his paper thus: "My attention has been increasingly directed toward a large group of women who are handicapped by premenstrual disturbances of manifold nature. It is well known that normal women suffer varying degrees of discomfort preceding the onset of menstruation. Employers of laborers take cognizance of this fact and make provisions for the temporary care of their employees. These minor disturbances include increased fatiguability, irritability, lack of concentration, and attacks of pain. In another group of patients, symptoms complained of are of sufficient gravity to require rest in bed for one or two days. In this group, particularly, pain plays the predominant role. There is still another class of patients in whom grave systemic disorders manifest themselves predominantly during the premenstrual period." The latter, he said, "complain of unrest, irritability, 'like jumping out of their skin,' and a desire to find relief by foolish and ill-considered actions. Their personal suffering is intense and manifests itself in many reckless and sometimes reprehensible actions. Not only do they realize their own suffering, but they feel conscience-stricken toward their husband and family, knowing well that they are unbearable in their attitude and their actions. Within an hour or two after the onset of the menstrual flow complete relief from both physical and mental tension occurs.'' He treated mild cases with diuretics, which brought some relief to those who retained fluids. In the more severe cases, he treated the women with radiation to the ovaries.

After the landmark Frank paper, another spate of research was published about conditions that recurred premenstrually: weight gain, fluid retention, ulcerative vulvitis, stomatitis, allergies, acne and dermatitis, irritability, restlessness, crying spells, headache, dizziness, insomnia, and painful breasts. In 1938 in a major article in the *Journal of the American Medical Association,* Leon Israel published a comprehensive article on ''The Premenstrual Tension,'' in which he detailed a spectrum of recurring symptoms, ascribed their cause to a deficiency of progesterone in relation to excess estrogen, and reported that progesterone was an effective therapy.

The following year, E.C. Hamblen, a prominent gynecologist at Duke University, published his textbook, *Endocrine Gynecology.* Omitting any mention of Frank's work and Israel's paper, Hamblen wrote, ''Despite the fact that menstruation is a physiologic process, most women experience certain subjective symptoms during the cycle... These include moderate lower abdominal discomfort, localized particularly in the pelvis; some slight mental depression; lassitude; a tendency to be annoyed readily; mild gastrointestinal symptoms...'' In a chapter on ''Abnormal Symptomatology of the Menstrual Cycle,'' Hamblen briefly described some symptoms that trouble women before menses, including premenstrual headaches, allergies, edema and fluid retention, skin disorders, breast discomfort, and psychoses. He did not categorize them as part of a common syndrome though.

The stream of publications continued. Researchers reported treating premenstrual tension marked by fluid retention with diuretics, premenstrual nervousness with progesterone injections, premenstrual tension as a nutritional deficiency with Vitamin B complex, and as hypoglycemia with a change in diet. In 1947 in the *Journal of Industrial Medicine,* Billig and Spaulding wrote about a ''frequent striking clinical syndrome in women consisting of a triad of symptoms: a burst of energy several days before menses (premenstrual tension, easy bruising, and lowered threshold to pain.) These patients, just prior to menses, feel the urge to do something such as cleaning the house, doing the laundry. They are hyper-irritable, crabby, and admit to being 'hard to live with.' Invariably, they will find black and blue marks on their bodies and often have no idea how they were incurred. Practically all of them are somewhat irritable and hypersensitive, and tend to flinch when someone touches them. There is usually a history of recurrent complaints of peripheral radicular pains, which is usually the presenting complaint. They will readily admit that they 'just can't stand pain.' In many, considerable domestic difficulties are present, and frequently, they are a serious problem. A fair percentage give a history of munching and nibbling in between meals, and of increased nervous tension when meals are missed or delayed. Yet a surprising number eat little breakfast, and it is primarily the noon meal and the afternoon snacks which they rely upon to 'make them feel better'...." Their study noted that glucose tolerance tests revealed these women were hypoglycemic prior to menstruation.

More articles followed. Again the researchers reported premenstrual hypoglycemia, fluid retention, edema, psychotic episodes, postpartum depression, and raised the possibility that the recurring premenstrual symptoms were linked to a deficiency of progesterone relative to estrogen. In 1953, Dr. Katharina Dalton, who was to come to the forefront in the diagnosis and treatment of premenstrual syndrome in England, published an article together with Raymond Greene entitled, "The Premenstrual Syndrome," in the *British Medical Journal*. They wrote, "The term 'premenstrual tension' is unsatisfactory, for tension is only one of the many components of the syndrome. Its use has commonly led to a failure to recognize the disorder when tension is absent or is overshadowed by a more serious complaint. We have preferred to use the term 'premenstrual syndrome' but as our investigation has progressed it has become clear that this term also is unsatisfactory. Though the syndrome most commonly occurs in the premenstrual phase, similar symptoms occasionally occur at the time of ovulation, in the early part of the menstrual phase, and even rarely in the first day or two after the flow has ceased. The term 'menstrual syndrome' though correct, for in each individual the symptoms recur at monthly intervals, may wrongly create the impression that they occur only at menstruation. We have finally decided to retain the term 'premenstrual syndrome' in the full realization of its imperfection. The full elucidation of its cause may later suggest a more appropriate and more accurate nomenclature."

The first symposium on premenstrual tension was published in November 1953 in the *International Record of Medicine,* edited by Joseph Morton. The articles covered the history, clinical pattern, psychological symptoms, treatment, impact on industry, and legal implications. The following year Katharina Dalton published an article in the *British Medical Journal* on PMS, toxemia in pregnancy, and progesterone therapy.

Unfortunately, most of the studies are flawed in some way, which makes it extremely difficult to draw conclusions about PMS. They lack the controls and the careful synchrony of standardized scientific research. Without such consistency, it is difficult to draw upon these studies to pinpoint the causes and patterns of the disorder. Many studies include heterogeneous groups of patients instead of patients grouped by similarity of symptoms. Patients whose only symptoms are profound depression with feelings of isolation, hopelessness, or suicidal intent should not be scrutinized alongside patients with no psychological symptoms. Some studies do not specify that the post-menstrual period must be symptom-free. Consequently, patients who have other disorders, such as clinical depression, which may worsen just prior to menstruation but appears throughout the cycle, may be mixed in with patients with PMS. Control groups should be matched for age, demographics, weight, and history of pregnancy.

The most exciting research theory about the cause of PMS is that proposed by Drs. Robert Reid and S.S.C. Yen, reported in an article in the *American Journal of Obstetrics and Gynecology* in 1981. They attribute the broad-based nature of premenstrual syndrome to the "abberrant release of, or sensitivity to" hormones in the hypothalamus — beta-endorphin and alpha-melanocyte stimulating hormones. This results in a cascade of changes in the neuro-endocrine systems — within the brain-hypothalamus-pituitary complex — that ultimately leading to the various manifestations of PMS. The regulation of neurotransmitters (biochemical messengers between cells in the brain) is controlled by neuropeptide hormones. (Beta-endorphin and alpha-melanocyte stimulating hormone are neuropeptide hormones.) When the normal balance of these hormones is disturbed, alterations in mood and behavior are produced. Also, the pituitary will release greater amounts of other hormones that may have a number of effects on the body, including changes in the estrogen/progesterone ratio, levels of prolactin, levels of vasopressin, and alterations in the effects of such substances as dopamine, epinephrine, and norepinephrine. Regulation of progesterone and estrogen in response to these changes differs from woman to woman and may account for the various clinical signs of PMS. Future research will tell us how accurate this sophisticated theory is.

SECTION II / *Shared Pain*

Chapter 3

"Migraine headaches were, as everyone who did not have them knew, imaginary. I fought migraine then, ignored the warnings it sent, went to school and later to work in spite of it, sat through lectures in Middle English and presentations to advertisers with involuntary tears running down the right side of my face, threw up in washrooms, stumbled home by instinct, emptied ice trays onto my bed and tried to freeze the pain in my right temple, wished only for a neurosurgeon who would do a lobotomy on house call, and cursed my imagination."

Joan Didion, **The White Album**

Migraine

"A razor blade embedded in the side of my head."

"A piercing, blinding weight, like a meteor that crashed down from the heavens directly onto my brain."

"An intense heat, as if all the blood vessels, veins, arteries in the right side of my head were engorged, slowly expanding over a matter of hours until my eye and the lobe of the brain behind it felt like they would explode. But the explosion never comes."

The migraine sensation intrudes into the consciousness in distinctive ways. It is unquestionably memorable, a kind of heinous torture that, once braved, finds its way into diaries, journals, letters to friends and families as if the victims pray to exorcise the migraine demon by extruding it in writing.

Menstrual migraine headaches are among the oldest recognized illnesses. First identified by Hippocrates, who attributed the symptoms to "agitated blood seeking a way of escape," they are severely disabling headaches that always recur at the same phase of the menstrual cycle. Migraine, whether associated with the menstrual cycle or not, is predominantly a women's illness. A study by a Scandinavian researcher, T. Dalsgaard-Nielsen, revealed that boys and girls aged seven to thirteen years had a similar incidence of migraine, but after the age of thirteen girls had a higher prevalence and more severe headaches than did boys; that suggests that the hormonal changes associated with menstruation increase susceptibility. Eighty percent of the migraine attacks are suffered by women. (Yet some of the most famous migraine victims are found in that remaining twenty percent: Thomas Jefferson and Ulysses S. Grant, among them.) Most women say that their headaches regularly strike at some point before or during their periods. Many women with premenstrual syndrome report menstrual migraine as one of their symptoms; about forty percent of our patients have a history of migraine.

The extensive research and literature about migraine has failed to isolate a single cause or develop a universal therapy for the blinding vascular headaches. What is known is that migraine, or the predisposition to it, is hereditary. For those who find no history of migraine in the family tree, the medical literature advises that there is a "migraine personality:" individuals who could be portrayed as ambitious, introverted, compulsive, highly organized, perfectionists intolerant of error. Type A workaholics have a disposition toward migraine. And a disparate range of incidents may act as catalysts: stress, fatigue, allergies, flashing lights, abrupt changes in pressure, humidity, or temperature, and of course, menstruation or ovulation.

The aura that precedes an actual migraine distracts and disrupts, results in clumsiness, accidents, oversights, incoherence. Migraine itself may be accompanied by nausea and vomiting, chills and bouts of sweating, exhaustion, distortion of vision or hearing, extreme sensitivity to all sensory stimuli. Many drugs and therapies are used to try to control migraine, but once an attack is under way, rarely does medication touch it.

Any or all of these symptoms and experiences may occur with a menstrual migraine. It most commonly appears just prior to the onset of the period or during the actual flow, but sometimes occurs mid-cycle at the time of ovulation. Very often the migraine seen with menses will disappear during pregnancy only to return following delivery; it often subsides with menopause. Like a bad penny that plagues the ill-starred, menstrual migraine tends to increase in frequency and intensity with age and multiple pregnancies. Many women who have had hysterectomies but still have their ovaries experience headaches every twenty-eight to thirty days or so, the kind of cyclical occurrence that women who have been sterilized report with other PMS symptoms.

Many of the women we've treated for PMS recall that their first migraine episodes were triggered by pregnancy. Vanessa Clayton is married and the mother of two children. After the birth of her first child nine years ago, she began to experience severe depression, irritability, outbursts of anger, and other symptoms. Her dominant symptom, however, was migraine so severe that the attacks lasted ten days at a time.

"I was in the hospital every month for a few days," she says, "The doctors did tests for a brain tumor and everything else. After not finding a brain tumor, they told me about the migraine personality and suggested that the stress of a new baby could cause it, and they sent me home with medication for migraine." Drugs had little effect on the migraine pain; after the birth of her second child, her attacks increased in frequency and severity.

"The headache always preceded my period by one day," she recalls. "I felt I was the opposite of catatonic. Catatonics don't respond to any stimulus. I responded to everything. Light bothered me. Noise drove me crazy. If someone touched me, I jumped. And smells made me nauseated. I needed a lot of salt and sugar to make things taste right. I remember lying on my bed, trying to be catatonic so the pain would stop. I would lie very still, wishing the pain away, trying to be the way I thought catatonics would be. Somehow it never made the pain go away." For nearly ten years, every month spelled a fresh migraine attack and an emergency trip to the university hospital for Vanessa Clayton. "Time didn't exist for me because I did nothing but lie in bed in pain for days on end. And then I would get up and would be functioning again.''

She tells a story of a typical incident that occurred after a migraine incident. ''Once I got my migraine and had to be taken to the hospital the day after I had picked up the laundry and dry cleaning for the family. I had picked up seventeen shirts for my husband, almost every one he owned. After I got home from the hospital, my husband came to me one morning and asked where his clean shirts were. I gave him a lecture about his inability to find anything in the house and sent him back to look for them. Then he came back again after not finding them, and I insisted that there were seventeen clean shirts that I had picked up from the laundry. At that, my husband said, 'Van, that was two weeks ago.' I had been totally unaware of how much time had passed since my migraine attack.

''That happened all the time. A sort of amnesia sets in with women with PMS. It's how we keep going each month. If you remembered it all, the pain, the fights, the terrible things you say to those you care about, and had to face it happening again to you, you wouldn't choose to live. So you forget. Conveniently. It's a defense mechanism. I would forget the pain. The problem, at the end, was that the pain dominated my existence, and I had only a few days of normalcy a month.''

In the three years before she came to our office, Mrs. Clayton's migraine and other symptoms lasted three weeks of the month. Since she's been on progesterone, changed her diet, and started to exercise regularly, her headaches are gone.

Another of our patients, Susan Henshaw, thirty-nine, also started having severe migraine headaches after the birth of her first child. The headaches would begin the day she began to menstruate, and last from two to six days. During those days, she would lie on her bed in a dark room. She saw neurologists, who took brain scans and prescribed ''every drug in the book.'' None of the standard migraine drugs worked. She was finally given Midrin, a combination of Tylenol and a mild sedative which is thought to contract the blood vessels in the brain. The Midrin relieved her headaches. Mrs. Henshaw, who says she would classify herself as a Type A/migraine personality, now realizes that the tension headache that built up during the premenstrual period culminated in a migraine. In the eighteen months that she has been treated with progesterone, and followed our prescribed lifestyle program, she, too, has been free of migraine.

Menstrual Headache

Migraine is not the only headache with a menstrual connection. All types of headache strike more frequently at some time in the menstrual cycle, say many researchers, including Dr. Katharina Dalton. Forty percent of our patients experience premenstrual headaches that are not migraine. Muscle-contraction headaches, marked by stiffness in the neck and the feeling of a tight, constrictive band around the head, sometimes accompany cyclical feelings of anxiety and irritability. Premenstrual symptoms such as irritability, weight gain, abdominal distention, and breast swelling and tenderness seem to be more prevalent in women who also suffer from any type of menstrually-related headaches.

But migraine, with its crippling, lengthy attacks, is the headache for which patients are most likely to seek medical help. Some studies attribute the cause of these attacks to hypoglycemia, tension, or water retention. In one study, Dr. Katharina Dalton analyzed the incidence of migraine and the eating patterns of more than two thousand women, and found that three-quarters of the participants were stricken by the headaches within twenty-four hours after they had eaten either chocolate, cheese, citrus fruits, or alcohol. Two-thirds of the women reported that they had fasted during the twenty-four hours before the attacks, having gone without food for five hours in the daytime or thirteen hours overnight. Her study indicated that careful attention to a hypoglycemic diet, with frequent small meals and an avoidance of salt, sugar, and alcohol, could have some effect in limiting migraine attacks.

One popular theory about menstrual migraine is that fluid retention plays a major role, which is why many women with migraine are encouraged to take diuretics and eliminate salt from their diet. This therapy doesn't alleviate the headaches completely but may modify the severity of the symptoms; we now know that only about thirty percent of women with premenstrual syndrome actually retain fluids so the investigations citing water retention as a major cause of menstrual migraine need to be re-examined.

Most migraine sufferers have tried half a dozen medications in their mission to end the pain. One preventive that works for some people is old-fashioned ergotamine tartrate, which constricts the swelling blood vessels during the "aura," the period of a few minutes or several hours that usually precedes the actual headache. Sometimes medications for migraine can be used intermittently at the time of menses in an effort to prevent the periodic occurrence of menstrual migraine. The most powerful weapons in the anti-migraine arsenal are methysergide, propranolol, and cyproheptadine, all of which may induce significant side effects for some people. (Methysergide is a derivative of lysergic acid; Sandoz Pharmaceuticals first synthesized LSD-25 while looking for a migraine cure.) But since the medications are used only intermittently for short periods of time in menstrual migraine, there is little need to fear using them.

Hormonal factors head the list of theories proposed about the cause of migraine, and are inextricably tied to the fluid retention theory. Water retention may be the result of an imbalance between estrogen and progesterone levels; falling estrogen levels in the premenstruum is probably the trigger mechanism in inducing menstrual migraine. Experiments have shown that it is possible to postpone the onset of migraine attack by introducing large amounts of estrogen into the bloodstream, by injection or oral intake. Migraine has occurred when researchers withdrew the estrogen support. Most women who suffer from premenstrual migraine notice that they are headache-free during pregnancy, especially during the last six months. Women who say their headaches are more severe during pregnancy are fewer in number. This strongly suggests that migraine is tied to the balance between estrogen and progesterone. Progesterone treatment is most effective in those women who suffer their headaches only at the time of the premenstrual phase of the cycle. It is next to most effective in those women who suffer from headaches at the time of premenstrual phase and during the time of their period. It is least effective with women who suffer headaches intermittently throughout the menstrual cycle but with increased frequency. Some women who take progesterone for PMS find that it is helpful for their headache during the time of the premenstrual phase; those who also have a history of headaches occuring during the menstrual period note that stopping the progesterone sometimes will cause a headache to occur during the ensuing menstrual period.

Premenstrual syndrome is not the cause of migraine, but migraine may be a symptom of the premenstrual condition. Progesterone is not a treatment for migraine per se, but may be helpful in treating premenstrual migraine, especially when the progesterone is taken in conjunction with an improvement in diet and exercise.

Chapter 4

*"Then suddenly it was as if a gulf
opened before him, and an extraordinary
inner light flooded his soul."*

Fyodor Dostoevsky, **The Idiot**

Epilepsy

When ancient healers began to observe a regular, periodic increase in epileptic seizures in women they naturally attributed the phenomenon to the moon, linking the two most common cyclical events of their experience. Since epilepsy was then adjudged a sign of madness and it was believed that insanity was intermittent, intensified when the moon was full, this led to the branding of epileptics (among others) as "lunatic," from the Latin word for moon.

As Fyodor Dostoevsky observed in his 19th Century novel *The Idiot,* "The sight of . . . an epileptic fit fills many with absolute and unbearable horror, which has even something mystical about it." The fear that surrounded these seizures, he pointed out, sprang from the frightful and apparently inexplicable changes in the victim's body, the distortion of the face and eyes, convulsions, and spasm that gripped the body vise-like and thrashed it mercilessly about, but most of all because "a terrible, incredible scream, unlike anything imaginable, breaks forth; and with this cry all resemblance to a human being seems suddenly to disappear."

Dostoevsky's powerful imagery emerged from an intimate knowledge of seizures; he himself was an epileptic.

The relationship between epilepsy and the menses was not explored scientifically until the last century, and even now medical researchers are just beginning to draw some conclusions about cyclical seizures. Perhaps the most important step for humankind that the scientists took was to cut all ties to the waxing and waning of the moon's phases. Instead of lunar seizures we have catamenial epilepsy, from the Greek word meaning monthly. Many researchers maintain that seizures are exacerbated by menstruation in about fifty percent of the women with epilepsy. In women with catamenial epilepsy, the seizures often begin, or pre-existing attacks recur or become worse at menarche. Menopause seems to have a significant depressant effect on the incidence of seizures. Catamenial seizures are not the only cyclical form of epilepsy. Rhythmic seizures in women, with a periodicity ranging from eight to forty-six days, were tracked in a 1955 study; other researchers have found monthly seizure patterns in men.

About ten percent of the patients we see have epilepsy or histories of seizures; practically all experience grand mal seizures marked by muscle spasms and lapses into unconsciousness. With the development of anticonvulsant drugs, scenes like those described by Dostoevsky are rare. Most of our patients are well-controlled with anticonvulsant drugs on a regular basis, but they frequently have disturbances just before their period. One of our patients responded well to Tegretol, an anticonvulsant, except that she noticed that if she had a seizure it was on the day of ovulation or the day her period started.

Britt Weston, a twenty-year-old college student, had the same kind of experience. Her cyclical symptoms began very early, when she was about eight, as she entered puberty, and continued through her teens. Four days a month she was fatigued, cranky, moody, and threw tantrums. "I'd be depressed and I wouldn't know why." She was examined by a neurologist, an internist, and an endocrinologist, none of whom could diagnose her disorder. They told her that it was all "in her head," and suggested that she see a psychiatrist. She wouldn't because "I knew that I wasn't crazy. I'd rather live with it than pay a doctor who won't cure it anyway. It would all disappear after four days." Weston had been treated for epilepsy, and was taking anticonvulsant medication. It prevented the attacks most of the time. If she were under unusual stress or became very excited or overtired, though, she sometimes had a grand mal seizure.

At the onset of menses her symptoms worsened. She saw a gynecologist who properly diagnosed her low blood-sugar level. Weston then went to see an internist, who put her in the hospital for further tests. The hospital's chief of medicine diagnosed her as "progesterone sensitive" and put her on birth control pills. She said that he called once a month to find out how the pills were working. Each month she told him that her symptoms were worse, not better, and he said, 'Just give it one more month.'" After five months, she just stopped taking them. "I'd have terrible mood swings and depression for about three or four days out of the month. I didn't know how it started, but once it did, I couldn't get out of it. I'd just have to wait, and ride it out. I could do just about everything that I had to if I didn't have a seizure. If I had a seizure, I'd get a terrible headache and I'd be too weak to do anything that day." Eventually she realized that the seizures occurred only when she was reacting to stress on the day of ovulation or three days before menstruation. During this time her family "just ignored it. Once they realized what it was, they'd just pretend it wasn't happening. It was the best thing to do. There's nothing they could have done for me anyway. No matter what they'd say, I'd scream and yell and cry. But only for four days." Progesterone has alleviated all of her symptoms.

"Every once in a while, if I forget to take the progesterone, I have problems. If I remember, I'm fine. I thought that I'd have to live with this for the rest of my life. It's a miracle."

Dr. Richard H. Mattson, professor of neurology at the Yale University School of Medicine and director of the Epilepsy Center at the Veterans' Administration Hospital in New Haven, Conn., is a leader in the field of epilepsy research. In a recently published study of fourteen women during three to six consecutive menstrual cycles, he concluded that seizures:

- Correlate with the stages of the menstrual cycle.
- Are most frequent at menstruation.
- Are most common when progesterone levels are lowest.
- Can be caused by stress independent of the menstrual cycle.

Until Dr. Mattson began his research, the studies done for catamenial epilepsy had been limited by insufficient controls and insufficient followup of the patients in the study. Other studies and clinical observations vary widely from Dr. Mattson's findings. This may in part be due to the lack of consistent definition of the catamenial phase. Some researchers consider it to be the last four premenstrual days and the first day of menstruation. Others limit it to the two days prior to the period and the entire duration of menstruation.

Hormonal Triggers

Estrogen and progesterone are at the center of the debate over the triggering mechanism of seizures. Both hormones have been used in experiments with animals and humans to determine their effect on seizure frequency. A 1976 Scandinavian study of seven women indicated a rise in the incidence of seizures when progesterone levels dropped — prior to menstruation — making estrogen more dominant. The study also showed a reduction in seizures when progesterone levels were higher. Laboratory tests using progesterone and some other related steroids produced anticonvulsive properties in animals. And a substance closely related to progesterone, desoxycorticosterone, exerts an anticonvulsant effect in epileptic persons. While the results are not conclusive, "estrogen seems to have some epileptic capacity and progesterone seems to have some anti-epileptic capacity," explains Dr. Allan Hauser, assistant professor of neurology and public health at Columbia University and assistant director of Columbia's Sergievsky Center for the study of epilepsy and cerebral palsy.

In a study of twenty-five women with epilepsy focusing on the role of estrogen in seizures, more than half were found to have menstrual problems — premenstrual syndrome or irregular menses. Their spells clustered during and immediately before menstruation. The study group were given Premarin, an estrogen, which activated their seizures. The predominance of estrogen in the body prior to menstruation suggests that it may cause catamenial epilepsy; that, in turn, suggests that progesterone, an antagonist of estrogen, could prevent attacks. We have found this to be true in the patients with a history of epilepsy whom we treat with progesterone for premenstrual syndrome.

Unfortunately most physicians and researchers do not seem to understand the distinction between progesterone and synthetic progestational agents. In our clinical practice we prescribe progesterone, a compound identical to the molecular structure of the progesterone produced by the ovaries, in treating PMS. This is the therapy that produces excellent results in treating PMS and its related symptoms. Most of the treatment and experiments in hormonal-related conditions in women involve the use of synthetic progestational agents (not progesterone) or oral contraceptives containing estrogen, which frequently exacerbate a range of PMS symptoms including epilepsy.

Epilepsy does not cause PMS, and PMS does not cause epilepsy. However, seizures may occur in some women premenstrually and may be part of the PMS spectrum of symptoms. We have seen some women who have been properly diagnosed and treated for their epilepsy whose seizures are controlled by medication — except during the premenstrual period. Progesterone has been an effective adjunct in the treatment of these premenstrual epileptic seizures.

Chapter 5

"Premenstrual tension produces this dichotomy, for while part of me feels lunatic, another me stands by appalled at what the premenstrual self is doing and saying. Or screaming, in this case..."

Brian Moore, I Am Mary Dunne

Mood Swings and Depression

On the morning of Caroline Lind's wedding day in 1970, she wandered about her parent's house, pausing over mementoes and photographs, saying farewell to the things of girlhood. In the playroom that had been her haven, she browsed among the toys and books shared among five brothers and sisters, finally reaching for a gently worn, well-thumbed copy of Hans Christian Andersen's *Fairy Tales*. She leafed through the volume until she came to her favorite story, "The Snow Queen," about two children, Gerda and Kay, and a demon's magic mirror. Central to the fable is "...that horrid mirror in which all good and great things reflected in it became small and mean, while the bad things were magnified and every flaw became very apparent." When the mirror breaks, grains of glass shower the earth, flying into people's eyes, and striking at their hearts. The little boy, Kay, is one of the unlucky victims who soon has no capacity for love, kindness, generosity, or the appreciation of beauty, and comes under the spell of the Snow Queen, who turns his heart to ice. As Caroline read, she recalls, "I realized that that was how I felt each month, as if the demon's mirror shattered and sent shards of glass into my eyes and my heart. I was two different people, the good person and the bad person. When I was feeling angry, irritable, depressed, and in pain, no one could do anything right, no one could say anything right to me, I couldn't accept kindness. I was belligerent, hostile, I'd throw things. I was just like little Kay.''

Caroline Lind is one of the many women whose premenstrual syndrome is marked by sharp mood swings and depression. More than half the women we treat indicate that they experience mood swings or depression in the phase between ovulation and menstrual flow as a PMS symptom; during the rest of their cycle, the behavior of these women is normal. Our patients quite spontaneously describe themselves as Dr. Jekyll and Mrs. Hyde, or as two opposite personalities inhabiting one body — the good person and the bad person, or the sane twin and the mad twin. These labels are not simply whimsical flights of fantasy. Dramatic changes in their behavior, moods, and personality are confirmed by husbands, children, close relatives, friends, roommates, and co-workers. While many of these women say they have an inward sense of being ''out of control,'' most do, in fact, control their behavior but fear that if the symptoms worsen they might assault their husbands or children. Very few women actually become violent. Verbal abuse, however, is common enough.

In some PMS women mood swings and depression develop slowly over several days; in others, the onset is very rapid. Self-esteem disintegrates with the inability to control the drastic shifts in personality and temperament, and the recurring sense of emotional helplessness. Most of our patients say they spent years berating themselves, asking ''what is wrong with me?'' or ''why don't I have the willpower to control this? or ''why I am different from other women?'' The only way to restore a woman's self-worth and confidence is to treat her premenstrual condition and any depressive disorder she may have, and reassure her that millions of other women share her feelings. Research studies also verify the preponderance of this type of behavior during the premenstrual phase, especially in the last four days prior to and the first four days of menstruation. It is manifested in the increase in female suicides, calls to psychiatric hotlines, appearances at psychiatric emergency facilities, admissions to hospitals for psychiatric and physical reasons, and crying spells.

Unhappiness vs. Depression

Like ''love'' and ''happiness,'' depression is as hard to qualify as it is to quantify. Unhappiness over disappointments or frustrations in everyday life confront everyone. Just because you're unhappy over not getting a promotion or because the washing machine is broken does not mean you're depressed. Unhappiness is distinguished from depression by the duration and pervasiveness of the mood. Depression is a persistent inability to experience pleasure or interest in *all* facets of life. If a woman lawyer loses a major court case and is still able to enjoy a game of tennis or dinner with friends at her favorite restaurant, if the low mood generated by her professional setback does not overshadow the rest of her life, and dissipates in a matter of days, she isn't depressed, just unhappy. Natural levels of the blues or brief bouts of feeling low strike most individuals at some point, whether they're ending a love affair or they've been fired from their job. But if you can't pull yourself together after a time and are unable to enjoy any facet of personal or work situations, you're suffering from depression.

The earmarks of depression — mood swings, the blues, unprovoked crying jags, fatigue, a sense of being out of control, distraction or a lack of concentration, lack of or sudden spurts of energy, lack of coordination, decreased sex drive — are among the most universal heralds of ovulation and menstruation. For most women these episodes are brief and disappear once menstruation begins. However, about thirty percent of the women burdened by extreme cases of PMS develop severe clinical depressions apart from the premenstrual disorder. Like storm clouds that hover above the horizon in the dog days of summer, shrouding the landscape in oppressive torpor, these depressions tinge every facet of daily life; they do not lift once menstrual flow starts. Women with major depressions must be treated both for their PMS and for the depressive condition.

If asked to name the single most common medical complaint of American women, in fact, many physicians would not hesitate in their response. An insidious, inward-directed anger, depression affects perhaps eighty-five percent of the female adults in this country at one time or another, according to some researchers' estimates. Most women do not even know they are depressed and do not seek medical treatment for the disorder, according to a study by Dr. Myrna Weissman, director of the Yale Depression Unit. Instead, they admit to bouts of feeling down, lethargic, unhappy, sad, gloomy, or troubled, but stumble along on their own and try to cope. While depression can develop apart from PMS, it is highly likely that a substantial portion of these women exhibit depression as a symptom of premenstrual syndrome. Both are silent diseases whose victims tend to keep their pain to themselves, ashamed or afraid or unaware that normal life is not a series of days or weeks filled with gloom and despair.

Many of the women we treat have been examined by psychiatrists who either did not recognize the premenstrual syndrome and misdiagnosed them as having a severe depression, or did not recognize that the women were suffering simultaneously from premenstrual syndrome *and* a severe depression. Psychotherapy, tranquilizers, and antidepressant drugs, especially the tricyclic antidepressants, Sinequan, Tofranil, Elavil, and Triavil, are the most common treatments in these cases. But rarely do they have any effect on premenstrual syndrome. An indication of the frequency of these treatments was revealed in a 1972 study, which reported that seventy percent of all individuals treated with psychotropic drugs were female.

The frequency with which the diagnosis of depression is made for women was attacked by Phyllis Chesler in her polemic, *Women and Madness,* and by some other researchers who argue that the numbers lie. Chesler's view is that the medical profession practices social and sexual discrimination in labeling women "depressed" when their behavior doesn't conform with societal expectations of women's roles. Maggie Scarf, in her best-selling work about women and depression, *Unfinished Business,* rigorously rejected the "numbers do lie" theory. Scarf concluded, "Women simply are more depressed, in the aggregate, than are men, in the aggregate. Beyond the shadow of a doubt."

The cause of depression is disputed. Classic psychoanalysis suggests that women's envy of men and their masculinity is at the root. "Menstrual or menopausal depression may, of course, be symptomatic of a psychological conflict," Paula Weideger points out in *Menstruation and Menopause.* "Menstrual depression has been related to a failure to conceive," notes Constance Berry and Frederick L. McGuire, "...as a woman's rejection of her femininity." Like Freud, Karl Menninger asserts that "the envy of the male cannot be repressed and serves to direct her hostility in two directions: she resents the more favored and envied males while secretly trying to emulate them, and at the same time she hates and would deny her own femaleness." Both Menninger and Freud suggest that woman's rage and envy, inevitably unleashed when she has "failed" to conceive, is uncontrollable at menstruation. Most women — and many men — reject this penis-envy argument.

Research into the causes of depression, however, has indicated that hormones may play a role in triggering the episodes. It may well be that the hormonal changes critical to the orchestration of the menstrual cycle spark the mood swings and depressed states.

Women who suffer from PMS and a major depression seem to respond best to drugs known as monoamine oxidase inhibitors, such as Nardil, or to lithium carbonate. Again, these two medications may ease the depression but they have little or no effect on the PMS. When depression is simply a manifestation of PMS, our usual treatment for PMS eliminates the depression. This treatment includes changes in nutrition, exercise, stress reduction techniques, vitamin therapy, and progesterone, which you will learn about later in this book.

Typical of the confusing combination of depression and PMS is the experience of Jennifer Anderson, a thirty-six-year-old probation officer. "I could handle the physical symptoms," she says. "But I couldn't handle the depression. About one day before my period I would flip out." Her symptoms progressively worsened, with the depression lasting more and more days each month. One gynecologist prescribed diuretics and told her that she was depressed because of fluid retention. She visited a nutritionist who put her on a hypoglycemic diet, and later tried acupuncture and hypnosis. Eventually she was examined by three psychiatrists, one of whom told her that "some of her depression was related to her period." The psychiatrists tried putting her on antidepressants, but the drugs made her feel worse. Finally, she says, "I went to a psychiatric hospital." She left work one Friday during lunch and committed herself. "I didn't even tell anyone where I was going." Her period started the next day and her depression lifted. "If only I could have held on for one more day," she says. She believes that a lot of the depression that women experience is suppressed rage. "Women aren't allowed to be enraged in our society. It isn't 'nice.' So women suppress a lot of their anger." Progesterone and improved nutrition have helped in her case. "I'm less depressed, fewer days, anyway. Now I feel that I can handle the depression."

Lori Weiner, the thirty-nine-year-old mother of two children who works as a customer service representative at a bank, had had mild PMS since puberty: irritability, depression, nervousness, backaches, headaches. After a tubal ligation three years ago, all the symptoms, particularly the depression, got much worse. Gynecologists prescribed Darvocet, birth control pills, and other drugs, none of which helped. Her doctors told her that she "had to live with it." She saw two psychiatrists, and the second told her that although the PMS wasn't the cause of her depression, it was a factor that probably increased its severity. She was hospitalized for depression for about three weeks. "I felt better, but not one hundred percent."

Women who suffer from PMS and a severe depression are the hardest to treat. While the two disorders may be interrelated, they must be treated separately. Some women won't accept that. They come to our office after having tried so many other treatments that they are frustrated and angry. By the time we see them, they are pinning all their hopes for a cure on PMS because they have heard it is treatable with progesterone. Progesterone is not a universal therapy; it can't solve all ills. We emphasize that in our evaluation sessions. Women with depression and severe premenstrual syndrome need progesterone, lifestyle changes, and psychotherapy or antidepressant drugs. Without the psychotherapy or antidepressants, progesterone won't ease the depression.

One patient, Sally Hunter, could not accept the fact that she had a severe depression rather than PMS. After nearly a year of discussions with Hunter and her husband, she finally agreed to at least see a psychiatrist. She insisted on visiting a biologically oriented psychiatrist because she put a lot of faith in biological causes of illness. When Hunter went for the initial evaluation she was skeptical. But she did agree to go for a second session, again, very skeptically. Finally Hunter accepted the diagnosis of depression and agreed to begin psychotherapy in earnest. We later got her children into family therapy, too, because they had begun to withdraw, apparently because of her frequent angry outbursts. We suspected that she had abused her daughter, although Hunter wouldn't discuss it. The girl was especially withdrawn and the mother felt extremely guilty about her. For months the children didn't believe her when she said "I'm better. It won't happen again." They needed a third party, the therapist, to convince them.

The pattern of premenstrual depression is so familiar that it is now part of the novelists' palette. Brian Moore, the author of *I Am Mary*

Dunne, a psychological study of insanity, says his recollections of the dramatic personality changes weathered by a close woman friend with PMS guided him in fashioning his novel about "a character on the brink of madness." He was searching for a protagonist with whom his audience would be able to "sympathize or identify. Then I thought about premenstrual tension. I decided to use premenstrual tension as my madness... I think that premenstrual depression is the most acceptable form of madness in our society."

> *"I opened the bag of chocolate chip cookies and ate two, for pleasure, or the memory of pleasure. I didn't like the taste; it made my palate heavy and dull. But I went on eating. It was a way of getting through this difficult time, this difficult walk."*
>
> Mary Gordon, **Final Payments**

Eating Disorders

Food is not merely one of life's necessities; like sex, food is a basic pleasure and comfort. Whether exultant and celebratory or frustrated, lonely, sad, or bored, we reach out — for companionship, friends, lovers, or if it's the best alternative, for food. A nation of immigrants, with memories of the privation and hunger that haunted our families in the old country a generation or two or three ago, America put plenty on a pedestal, along with truth, justice, and opportunity. We once considered a groaning table a right of citizenship, conferred upon us for having shrewdly chosen to live in the world's bread basket, the land of amber waves of grain and coast-to-coast herds of dairy cows and beef cattle. Despite the trend in the last decade toward fitness and dieting, Americans continue to use and abuse food daily to a degree almost unchallenged, with the possible exception of Henry VIII. Our obsession with food, and sweets, in particular, starts in childhood with heavily sugared baby foods. From there we gavotte to the playground, filling ourselves with empty calories and energy bursts from the candy store. As Alfred Kazin, in *A Walker in the City,* recalls his own Depression-era childhood in New York, "We never had a chance to know what hunger meant. At home we nibbled all day long as a matter of course. On the block we gorged ourselves continually on 'Nestles,' gumdrops, poppy seeds, nuts, chocolate-covered cherries, charlotte russe, and ice cream... The hunger for sweets, jellies, and soda water raged in us like a disease; during the grimmest punchball game, in the middle of a fist fight, we would dash to the candy store to get down two-cent blocks of chocolate and 'small' three-cent glasses of cherry soda; or calling 'upstairs' from the street, would have flung to us, or carefully hoisted down at the end of a clothesline, thick slices of rye bread smeared with chicken fat.''

These days there's little of the chicken fat smeared on rye. Instead there's fast-food roulette. The ticky-tacky vista of red roofs, orange tiles, and Golden Arches that stretches along highway after highway the length and breadth of this country offers eloquent testimony to the fact that Americans don't eat well, they eat a lot. Television commercials and supermarket aisles repeat the message, this time with a parade of sugared cereals, ice cream, pudding, cakes, pies, and candy, alongside boxes and cans of heavily salted, sugared, floured, virtually sedated foods that can be fixed in a jiffy. Thirty million Americans may jog or participate in sports, but not all thirty million of them are living on spinach salads and fresh vegetables. If they were, the market for some of these instant carbo-caloric wonders would dry up.

This environment is a mined and dangerous trail for those receiving hunger signals from their brain. We know that depression and obesity may be due in part to an over-release of certain chemicals that act on the brain's hunger response, distorting an individual's response to and perception of food, and sometimes triggering cravings. Depression and food cravings recur regularly in many women with premenstrual syndrome. This may be a result of the hormonal balance in the body, but more research remains to be done — on PMS, depression, and food disorders — before the answers are known.

Eating Binges

Dr. Hilde Bruch, in her book *Eating Disorders,* says binge eating — the sudden, compulsive ingestion of very large amounts of food in a very short time, sometimes furtive, sometimes public — is usually triggered by stress or by feelings of loneliness, frustration, anxiety, tension, or boredom, or is a symptom of an underlying emotional illness, such as depression. It is extremely common among women, a significant percentage of whom are also depressed. She writes, ''...eating binges, uncontrolled eating in response to the slightest insult or disappointment, have occurred at some time or another in practically all of my fat patients." And the binges are almost always followed by self-recriminations.

Food binges wreak havoc, however temporary, in the lives of millions of women who can't control their cravings or attitudes toward food. Not surprisingly, the drama and destruction of binges can be found in fictional characters, too. In Mary Gordon's novel, *Final Payments*, the heroine Isabel Moore, reaches out for food in the midst of a depression following her father's death and her own search for identity. "I would eat later, secretly in my room. I hid a box of crackers under my bathrobe and went upstairs. I did not lift up the dark green shade. I put crackers in my mouth whole, and ate them silently, as if I were in a fever, as if I were being watched." In another instance: "I took off my clothes and got into bed in my bra and underpants. I had kept two bars of candy in my handbag. I ate them now, under the gray blankets." The emotional and physical effects of the binges were devastating. After a humiliating shopping trip to a dress store, she says, "Size sixteen, I kept saying to myself. But what did it mean? Ten, sixteen, my body had caused only damage... My thighs chafed against each other as I walked. I decided to go on a diet."

Bruch observes that for many "obesity has an important positive function; it is a compensatory mechanism in a frustrating and stressful life. In others, however, it is associated with, and directly related to, severe personality and developmental disturbances." Many people, she says, hide their emotional problems "under a complacent facade... Instead of expressing anger, or even experiencing it, they become depressed and the overeating serves as a defense against deeper depression... Overeating may occur at times of such severe emotional stress that the question is not so much 'Why overeating?' but 'What would be the alternative?'" She notes that statistics show that obese people have a higher incidence of most diseases and a higher death rate, but their suicide rate is dramatically lower. "I have often been impressed with the fact that the situations in reaction to which obesity developed were situations to which others might have reacted with despair," she notes. "However much of a handicap obesity may become, as a defensive reaction it is less destructive than suicide or paralyzing deep depression."

Cravings for food, but especially for chocolate, sweets, or salty foods, are frequently experienced by women with premenstrual syndrome — sometimes for an afternoon, sometimes for several days or more. When the cravings are strong, they result in binge eating. The women eat compulsively and are incapable of stopping themselves. It's not simply a matter of self-control; it's PMS. The physiology of the symptoms can't be controlled simply by wishful thinking. When women of normal weight and normal eating patterns binge briefly, they usually lose the extra four or five pounds once their period begins. Some women gain eight to fifteen pounds by binging and eventually have great difficulty losing this weight during their symptom-free portion of the month. It is not surprising to find then, that most women who have PMS are overweight, and at least seventy-five to eighty percent of these women binge. Women with PMS frequently have great fluctuations in weight during their adult years. Of the patients we see, about twenty percent are more than twenty-five pounds overweight; the majority are ten to fifteen pounds overweight. Many who binge as a result of PMS find that over time they can't control their eating patterns at all; they chronically overeat and may gain more than twenty-five pounds.

Lois Benson, one of our patients, remembers her experience with cravings before her period: "They would come about four or five days before. I would eat things that I wouldn't even look at ordinarily, and gain anywhere from ten to fifteen pounds. But I would lose ten of that a week after." Now treated with progesterone and following our nutritional program, she occasionally has one day of craving, but has lost ten pounds already and is continuing to lose weight.

Erin Gibson, forty-three, a journalist and mother of five, had regular, strong food cravings that led her to consume gallons of ice cream, bags of snack foods, and entire cakes over two or three days. Since starting progesterone therapy, her food cravings are reduced: "I'll eat a few handfuls of potato chips compulsively instead of the whole bag, half a pint of ice cream instead of a quart."

Marsha Coleman, thirty-seven, an investment counselor and mother of four, says her "abnormal craving for sweets started with ovulation. I used to put on five, six, seven pounds a month. My normal weight was about 130, but now I'm 120 and I don't lose from there, I don't gain from there. I have leveled off and I don't change weight at all, with or without my period. I had literally two sets of clothes. I always had to wear wraparound skirts at the end of the month."

Both Agnes Lazarus and her daughter, Deborah, were compulsive eaters until they began treatment for premenstrual syndrome. Mrs. Lazarus has lost fifteen pounds. She says the progesterone treatment has been important in improving her college-aged daughter's self-image. "Deb couldn't control her eating habits before. Now her depression is relieved and she has been able to stay on a diet for the first time in her life and lose weight."

Links between food cravings and menstruation, and cravings and depression have been studied by many scientific researchers. One study, by Stuart Smith and Cynthia Sauder, reported in *Psychomatic Medicine,* of three hundred nurses and a pilot study of thirty-seven hospitalized depressive patients, found that of the group of depressed patients, fifteen women, or more than forty percent, said they felt like eating compulsively prior to menstruation, and nine of those fifteen women, or twenty-four percent, reported experiencing premenstrual depression. Of the sixteen who said they craved sweets, twelve patients, or seventy-five percent, said they suffered from premenstrual depression. All nine who craved chocolate had premenstrual depression.

Sixty-six percent of the three hundred nurses studied said they were tense or depressed just before or at the start of their periods. The nurses' study also showed "a rather striking association between recurrent depression, premenstrual fluid retention, and a peculiar craving for sweets in the immediate predepressive and premenstrual period." Of the one hundred sixteen who reported a desire to eat compulsively at specific times, eighty-five, or seventy-three percent, said they had premenstrual tension or depression; of the sixty-four who said they craved sweets at specific times, forty-nine, or seventy-seven percent, said they had premenstrual tension or depression. Of the forty-two who craved chocolate at specific times, thirty-four, or eighty-one percent, reported premenstrual tension or depression. The premise of the Smith and Sauder study was their observation of three depressed female patients "who demonstrated a peculiar and characteristic craving for sweets" before their periods that was "not present under normal circumstances. These persons did not normally tend to eat compulsively nor were they obese. Just prior to a period of depression, however, they reported a very powerful craving for sweets and in particular for chocolate, which they went to great lengths to obtain." Later they examined two younger patients with a craving for sweets "during the onset of depression." These women had considerable feelings of tension or depression just prior to the onset of each menstrual period and tended to retain large amounts of fluids then. They often developed a peculiar craving for sweets in the premenstruum."

Another investigation studied forty-five women, including twenty-five with premenstrual symptoms, who reported symptoms of irritability, fatigue, depression, crying spells, impatience, and cravings for sweets. Still another researcher, Joseph Morton, reported an alteration in carbohydrate metabolism to permit increased sugar tolerance. "The hypoglycemia is a recent and striking finding in premenstrual tension. It is clinically manifested by increased appetite or a craving for sweets." In Morton's study, thirty-seven percent of the women with premenstrual syndrome had cravings for sweets, and twenty-three percent had increased appetite. Tests of the women with premenstrual tension showed that they were hypoglycemic prior to the onset of their periods.

Anorexia Nervosa

About ten percent of the patients we see who are in their twenties and thirties have recovered from adolescent episodes of anorexia nervosa or bulimia, two eating disorders. Anorexics sometimes start by dieting from a slightly overweight or normal level with a goal of ten or more pounds under what would be an ideal weight; when they reach that level, though, they keep on dieting, refusing meals, balking at their favorite foods until their weight plunges to 90, 80, sometimes 70 pounds or less. Estimates of the incidence of anorexia range from one in one hundred adolescent girls to one in two hundred. Bulimics appear normal in appearance, usually maintaining an ideal weight. But they accomplish this through a bizarre pattern of binges and purges, much like the elite of Rome during a ritual feast. It is much more difficult to estimate the incidence of bulimia because frequently there are no outward symptoms; it's extremely common among high school and college students.

Women and girls trapped by these conditions have a distorted view of their own self-image and of food itself. Dr. Hilde Bruch, in *Eating Disorders,* defines the underlying personal feelings of anorexics as a "disturbance of delusional proportions in the body image and body concept." The anorexic seems to be completely unaware of her actual weight and size, insisting to her parents and friends that she is fat when she is actually little more than a walking, talking bag of bones. Dr. Bruch says some anorexics pursue thinness "in the struggle for an independent identity, delusional denial of thinness, preoccupation with food, hyperactivity, and striving for perfection." It is the ultimate, self-selected malady for a teenager unable to confront her emerging maturity. For an adolescent plagued by the pain and emotional turmoil of PMS on top of the identity crisis of youth, anorexia may be a comforting distraction, requiring concentration, willpower, and discipline; anorexic girls frequently come from an extremely close family and are "the perfect" daughters, who earn high grades in school and are usually very obedient. Anorexia is usually their only form of rebellion. Mara Selvini Palazzoli says a girl with this condition "believes that her mind transcends her body and that it grants her unlimited power over her own behavior and that of others... The result... is the mistaken belief that the patient is engaged in a victorious battle on two fronts" against her body and her family. In *The Art of Starvation*, Sheila MacLeod variously describes her schoolgirl experience with anorexia as "a form of passive resistance," and "my only weapon in my bid for autonomy." Her war was waged in response to the realization that "What was happening to my body — not only the changes brought about by puberty, but the fact that the clothes it wore and the food it consumed were chosen for it by someone else — was a metaphor for what was happening to me as a whole person."

When we see these women, food disorders are no longer a problem for them. Anorexics, whose percentage of body fat to body mass falls to a level below that necessary for menstruation, usually stop menstruating at some point in their weight loss or experience amenorrhea. Amenorrhea, we know, may act as a triggering event for premenstrual syndrome. Some of the former anorexics we see have recalled that they had cyclical symptoms prior to menstruation during their active anorexic phase. Others don't remember, but it appears that the PMS did not develop until after the anorexia was under control. The connection between premenstrual syndrome and the incidence of anorexia and bulimia needs to be explored in formal research.

"I set some arbitrary rules for myself. I wouldn't drink until 5 p.m. I wouldn't drink before leaving the house to go shopping. I would drink only on alternate days. For months I made myself crazy, adhering to these self-imposed restrictions."

Joyce Rebeta-Burditt, **The Cracker Factory**

Problems With Alcohol and Drugs

Premenstrual syndrome gives many women more than enough reason to seek out liquor or other drugs to block out the pain, the depression, the memories of bizarre episodes with their families or at work. Compounding this cyclical tendency to reach for a drink, most women have a reduced tolerance for alcohol or drugs premenstrually — sometimes a dramatically lower threshold for these substances. Many women who normally consume two or three cocktails without incident find they become thoroughly intoxicated with one during the premenstrual phase. Like food binges, drinking sprees can be habit-forming. Once a woman starts drinking because of her PMS symptoms she may just keep on drinking all month long. Sandra Thomas, one of our patients, says, "I drank a lot during my premenstrual time to alleviate the symptoms. The trouble with drinking heavily for half the month is that you get into the habit. I started to drink just as heavily when I felt good as when I felt bad."

Women who drink or abuse drugs were, like women with PMS, once silent sufferers. No longer. Their problems and experiences have filled novels and autobiographies, movies, and television over the past decade. Perhaps the best story of the journey of a woman drinker from mental hospital to recovery is told in *The Cracker Factory,* the best-selling novel by Joyce Rebeta-Burditt. The heroine is Cassie Barrett, a woman with a history of major depressions and alcoholic episodes that have landed her in an institution twice. In the first eighteen pages and within just about as many days, we learn that Cassie:

- burns a dinner,
- has a car accident involving her children,
- throws another piping hot meal down the garbage disposal in the mistaken belief that she has already fed her family,
- is accused by her husband of being incompetent when she can't keep up with the laundry — forcing him to wear one brown and one black sock to work — and stashes the ironing overflow in shopping bags behind the furnace,
- and collapses in tears at a supermarket after staring blankly at the shelves, distracted and confused, not remembering what she came in to buy.

All of this has happened, we discover, because after a lengthy drying out period and stay in a hospital, Cassie has had it. "I grabbed my coat and the grocery money and was waiting at the liquor store when it opened... Once home I pulled the curtains, put on a stack of records and curled up in front of the stereo with a tumbler full of scotch. I sipped and listened and sipped some more, until the barbed wire dissolved and a soft, mellow fog replaced the ache behind my eyes. I must have fallen asleep because the next thing I knew the kids were home and Charlie was due. I knew I'd have to scramble frantically to get to the market and home again, get dinner started and some of the clutter cleared away before he walked in the door. But first I needed a drink."

It's a graphic, if nearly breathless, first chapter. But it does more than simply draw the reader into the book. It paints a picture of life for a lot of women, women who drink, women who are on pills, women who are depressed. Even women who have extreme cases of premenstrual syndrome. The one thing we don't know about Cassie is whether her problems are cyclical. Cassie does relate a brief family history in which she recalls the outbursts of Aunt Lily who threw the Thanksgiving turkey at Cassie's father because no one passed her the gravy, and set fire to the broom closet because the family didn't want to discuss Catherine the Great. PMS, like alcoholism and some psychological disorders, does run in families, as we explain in the following chapter.

Alcohol is a mood altering drug; it is a depressant, not a stimulant. For someone who is already depressed, alcohol fuels their despair and sense of hopelessness. In combination with any medication, alcohol's effects are magnified. Drugs and alcohol is a lethal combination. Yet after the age of forty, women rarely limit their abuse to alcohol alone, but tend to use a combination of drugs and drink.

Women and Alcohol

For as long as grape and grain have been fermented into potable liquids, some women as well as men have over-indulged. But society's traditional view of women did not leave room for weakness or illness; women were stuck on a plaster pedestal, expected to remain pure and prim, virgin or mother until they died. Reality, of course, never quite matched that portrait. Until fairly recently, though, women with drinking problems kept them hidden behind drawn curtains; for if the problem did become publicly known, they were shunned by the community. Women who drank were automatically thought to be "loose," or immoral, beyond the pale, Blanche DuBois in the flesh. Two developments helped millions of women leave the cooking sherry in the kitchen and seek help: the recognition in the 1960s that alcoholism is a disease, and the deluge of women into the workforce. At least one-third of the ten million alcoholics and problem drinkers in the United States, or 3.3 million, are women, according to *The Invisible Alcoholics* by Marian Sandmaier. Other estimates put the figure as high as one-half of problem drinkers, or five million women. The percentage of women in Alcoholics Anonymous has risen from twenty-two percent in 1968 to twenty-nine percent in 1977, with women comprising thirty-two percent of new members joining AA between 1974 and 1977. Sadly, the rise in the number of working women that made it impossible for many with drinking problems to ignore their weakness for liquor any longer, is also thought to have contributed to a further increase in women alcoholics. Stress is a critical factor in problem drinking, just as it is with premenstrual syndrome. The stress of a job, on top of the burden of maintaining home and family, can lead some women to liquor. "Women in the workforce drink more, and there are more women who work using drink and drugs than those who stay at home," says Dr. Michael Murphy, president of the Bay Area Comprehensive Alcoholic Program, which operates several treatment centers in the Boston area providing comprehensive alcoholic treatment to one thousand to two thousand outpatients a year. Sixty percent of those patients are women. In addition, BayCAP helps treat three hundred to four hundred women admitted to hospitals for treatment. Dr. Murphy says the danger signals for a chronic alcoholic, the stresses that trigger drinking, are feelings of anger, tiredness, loneliness, hunger, migraine headaches — all of which may be symptoms of premenstrual syndrome.

Of the patients we treat for premenstrual syndrome, about twenty percent abuse alcohol and fifteen percent belong to Alcoholics Anonymous, usually joining because we've referred them. About forty percent of our patients are on some sort of medication when they come to our office. Valium and amphetamines are the most common. Valium is a tranquilizer, a muscle relaxant that induces a mild euphoria and is prescribed for anxiety; some of our patients have used as much as thirty milligrams a day or more; amphetamines, or speed, are an appetite suppressant and energy booster that helps some people temporarily cope with fatigue or depression. And we've treated one woman who had been a heroin addict; that extreme is rare.

Rita Hirsh's story is typical. Hirsh, a thirty-nine-year-old real estate broker, is married and has two sons. She began to drink after her PMS symptoms appeared to try to blank them out. "For two weeks, I would drink at home, quietly and alone. I wouldn't drink much when I was out. I had a very high tolerance for alcohol. There is no occasion that I can remember, or anyone I know can recall, when I acted drunk. When I first began attending Alcoholics Anonymous, many of my friends were surprised." Eventually she lost her capacity and tolerance for alcohol and began to have blackouts. Her first blackout occurred at a friend's house, where she and her family went for dinner. "I remember helping prepare dinner — pork curry. We sat down for dinner at eight, and I have no recollection of what happened after that. I don't remember what we talked about, I don't remember leaving with my kids at ten, putting them to bed, putting myself to bed. It's time lost forever. I got up the next morning and I had no memory of what happened the night before." The second time, she was home with her children. Her usual pattern, she said, was: "I'd pour myself a large glass of wine when I got into the house at five or six, and I'd drink slowly and steadily until I went to bed."

Her husband, Kenneth, didn't confront her with her alcoholism, even though he recognized it, because he thought it would destroy their marriage. "Now it's all to her credit that she recognized her problem and cured herself," he says. He noticed that she was drinking, but "we've always lived in a drinking environment. Drinks can close off your mind. I'd say to myself 'she's trying to block out the fight we're having.' When we fight, I tend to stop drinking. I think I'm afraid that I'd lose my temper. I did twice, in sports, and I really hurt people." (He is 6'3" and 220 pounds. Rita is 5'6" and 110 pounds.)

Hirsh says she was never noticeably drunk. Her husband remembers otherwise, especially the night that she threw a platter of prime rib against the dining room wall during a dinner party. Another major episode that occurred shortly before she decided to join AA, he says, came after they had had a major argument and she was particularly tense and angry. She told him she was going to get "as drunk as humanly possible." When she stomped upstairs during the fight, Kenneth Hirsh cleared all the liquor out of the house, packed up the children, and left. But he didn't see a bottle of wine and a gallon of vodka that were sitting on a kitchen counter. He says that leaving the liquor on the counter was "the biggest accident of my life, because she felt that I wanted her to drink herself to death." When he came home, "she was crying to her mother on the phone like a baby, then she got on with her father and I listened to her accuse him of never loving her or supporting her. When her friend finally came over and nurtured her, I left. Else I knew we would have a royal battle." The Hirshes began seeing a marriage counselor once Rita started progesterone therapy at the clinic; she also continues to attend AA meetings. "I'm an alcoholic. That means that I can't have one or two drinks ever, anymore," she says.

When Hirsh attended her first AA meeting, "I saw people like me. I heard many of the women speak of menstrual problems. There's a high incidence of PMS among women alcoholics, and a high incidence of alcoholism among women with PMS." Hirsh hesitated to tell her children about her alcoholism. "I went to AA meetings for two months before I told them. They noticed that I didn't drink anymore." She didn't tell them that she had stopped drinking, but "I knew that they knew. My husband would have wine with dinner, and I'd have ginger ale. They didn't question me, but I felt uncomfortable because I'm generally very open with them." She finally told her sons that she had an "allergy to alcohol," something that she felt they could relate to. She was attending AA meetings two or three times a week. First she told the boys that she was going to a "getting better" group. Finally she told them what it was. She was afraid, she said, that they'd find out from someone else.

Family Ties and Drinking Problems

Alcoholism runs in families; studies in this country and in Denmark have revealed a very strong genetic disposition to problem drinking. But men are more likely to become alcoholics based on genetic disposition, while females are more likely to show it as an effect of stress-related illness, like PMS, Dr. Murphy says. Many of our patients say their mothers, sisters, grandmothers or other female relatives drank because of what seemed to be a cyclical, PMS problem. Sometimes even children start drinking in reaction to a mother with PMS.

Carmen Sanchez, thirty-one, is an administrative assistant; she's married and the mother of a toddler. She is emphatic in her attitude to liquor: she doesn't drink and doesn't permit liquor in her home. Sanchez has had the symptoms of premenstrual syndrome since she began menstruating. She believes that PMS is the reason for the heavy drinking of her mother, grandmother, and sister. "My mother would drink very heavily the week before her period and get violent; she would beat my brother and me. For two or three weeks my mother would be fine, and then one week we all instinctively knew as very young children that something was wrong with her. My father would always say that mother was having her change this week. We got to notice the pattern... I think my mother's mother also has it. And my sister, too. I think it runs in the family. I can see it in just about every female member of my family, especially with its relation to the alcohol abuse. That's why I never drank. My sister was in the hospital about two months ago for thirty days. She had overdosed on alcohol somehow and her period was due in two days. My grandmother still says she has symptoms of PMS. She's a recovered alcoholic and lives in a nursing home. They're forbidden to have any kind of alcohol at all. She would say that she would always drink before her period because she couldn't deal with it. She's very outspoken about it, she talks about it a lot. She's eighty-three and she's still here."

Another patient, Gerry Simpson, also abstains from alcohol. Her mother had PMS and both parents were alcoholics. "My mother suffered rather severely from PMS when I was growing up, at least I now believe that. As a result, her marriage to my father was rocky and tumultuous. They both began to drink a lot. I think it was really as a result of my father's horrendous experience in the war (World War II) and my mother's PMS. I think they had started drinking to kind of overcome what had become an empty life." Simpson remembers: "My father's response to being drunk was to become violent and the first stage of my mother's nighttime ritual was to be verbally abusive, and then she would fall into a stupor. I was the caretaker of my family as we were growing up. My parents went through these alcoholic nightmares every night, but my older sisters and brother and my two little brothers slept through the violence and the nightmare. My father used to beat my mother regularly. My response to that was to get out of my bed and go and try to intervene in the conflict. I always did and I always succeeded; I was only nine or ten years old. I remember literally saving my mother's life on many occasions and putting them both to bed. Sometimes they would be totally unclothed, things would be bashed and broken all over the house. I remember really hating my brother and sister for not helping me through that. Eighty-five percent of the physical violence in that house was PMS-related, I'm sure. My mother would give everyone terrible verbal thrashings. I used to think that she was a witch; I thought she might have been possessed. I almost felt responsible for her tantrums because I knew she didn't like me. What really frightened me was taking on the characteristics of my mother, later. Of course, when I learned about PMS, I knew why my parents had had problems. She had PMS. It was why they were violent. Why she was alcoholic. Probably why he was an alcoholic."

The pattern of both husband and wife becoming alcoholics is not uncommon; in a relationship where the woman has premenstrual syndrome, her cyclical irritability and outbursts may trigger his drinking. After we presented material about PMS to a group of alcohol abuse therapists, one of the counselors said he had been confounded by the behavior of several men he was treating but now he recognized a pattern. "They have really worked hard in AA but every four to six months they start drinking again. And I've never been able to figure out why; they can't either. I know some of these guys' wives well enough and it's clear they've got PMS. I think when things have built up between the two of them over four or five months, then the wife has a severe episode of PMS, that's a crisis situation and the man deals with it by drinking." Since that discussion the counselor and several of his colleagues have referred the wives of their patients to us for treatment. Their diagnosis in these instances has been on target: the women have severe premenstrual syndrome.

We refer our patients with these problems to drug and alcohol abuse programs, especially Alcoholics Anonymous. Lifestyle changes and progesterone therapy are important in treating their PMS, but will not go to the source of their problems with alcohol. Progesterone may make it easier for some women to respond to treatment for alcohol and drug abuse because it tends to eliminate cyclical depression, anxiety, irritability — the kinds of problems that led them to alcohol and pills in the first place.

Chapter 8

"The lines are fallen unto me in pleasant places; yea, I have a goodly heritage."

Psalms, 16:6

It Runs in Families

Just as a droll wit or stubborn streak may pass from generation to generation in some families as predictably as great-grandmother's silver, a lineal disposition to health conditions is extremely common. Premenstrual syndrome appears to be one more characteristic that transcends generations. But it's hardly a tie that binds; PMS is more like an ineluctable fetter. We know that it runs in families. Once women are diagnosed and begin to understand the pattern of PMS, they rush to tell us stories about the troubles of their mothers, grandmothers, sisters, cousins, and aunts; more than half of our patients report that another family member has PMS. Like sure-fingered veterans at a quilting bee, they piece together incidents that strained family life and relationships and find that what had seemed to be the erratic or hostile behavior of a relative was classic premenstrual syndrome.

What we don't know yet is whether PMS is hereditary, if a genetic code is stamped on a woman's cells like electronic circuits etched on a silicon chip, programming her female descendants with the hallmarks of the syndrome. We've gathered some strong evidence that it might be. Several sets of twins have been treated at our center; in these cases, both women have the same symptoms and both experienced the same time of onset, whether at puberty or later. We have yet to find a twin who has PMS with a twin sister who does not. Dr. Katharina Dalton in England has made the same observation about PMS and twins. Many of our patients are mothers of twins but in most instances the children are too young to have developed PMS.

Genetic predisposition to the illness may be one reason or the entire reason that many women exhibit PMS at puberty. Or there could be a genetic predisposition that must be magnified by risk factors before the time bomb of the syndrome explodes in the system. Let's say your mother, grandmother, and sister have the symptoms, but you have never used the Pill, become pregnant, undergone a tubal ligation or hysterectomy, and avoided other risk factors. You may never develop PMS because, while you have a genetic predisposition to it, you have avoided the risk factors that would activate the signal in your genes.

Some scientists might argue that premenstrual syndrome is not hereditary, that it appears in relatives and close friends unconsciously. If A has premenstrual syndrome, and A lives with her mother and sister, B and C, works with D and E, and is extremely close friends with F, does the fact that A, B and C exhibit the same symptoms mean that the condition is genetic? Not necessarily. And what if you find that all of them — A, B, C, D, E, and F — have premenstrual syndrome? If it's genetically transmitted, then what's the explanation for its appearance in unrelated women? Could all these women from unrelated families experience the same genetic trait? We concede that there could be a role-modeling or mimic factor with the syndrome. To some degree, at least. Nonetheless, the frequency of the condition within families seems too high to be merely a coincidence or a copycat phenomenon.

The question of genetics can be answered once researchers devote the time and effort necessary to identify the genetic markers of PMS and trace them through many generations of families.

Searching Through the Family Tree

Our patients sometimes combine the analytical skills of Nero Wolfe and the practiced eye of a jigsaw puzzle fanatic in their efforts to hang PMS on the appropriate limbs of their family trees.

Barbara Southern, forty-six, and her twenty-two-year-old daughter, Holly, both are being treated at our Massachusetts center; Mrs. Southern's sister also has PMS, and their mother may also have suffered from it. Mrs. Southern feels that she probably had it during her teen years, but didn't connect it with her menstrual cycle until she reached her twenties. Her symptoms have changed over the years, initially encompassing depression, irritability, joint pains, back pains, compulsive eating binges, and fluid retention. "Depression used to be one of my biggest problems," she says. "It's gotten worse as I've gotten older." For the past eight years she has had a "peculiar stomach problem," which starts as hunger and becomes severe pain. "I have been trying [to find medical help] for years," she says.

She, perhaps understandably, was much more willing to discuss the depressive aspect of her daughter's PMS than her own. She says Holly's symptoms are like her own when she was younger: hunger, compulsive eating, binging, and serious depression. "I've always noticed it. It was very obvious — to me, not to Holly — when the second half of her cycle was beginning." Holly has thought of suicide during PMS and can't control her eating habits. Mrs. Southern said the long-distance telephone bills from her daughter, who's away at college, are heavy from mid-month on. "It's very difficult. I've seen it in her since she started her periods. No one would agree with me. But what could I do? I didn't even know how to help myself." Mrs. Southern says Holly has responded well to the progesterone therapy and lifestyle changes. "I'm in touch with her constantly. The depression is relieved. And she has been able to stay on a diet and lose weight.

"My sister has it, too. It seems to have gotten worse since she had a baby and two miscarriages. Of course, it's not as devastating for her. But she does report the fatigue, depression, and mood swings. Now my mother thinks she may have had symptoms of it, too."

Holly remembers that during her childhood her mother was frequently ill. "When I was a little girl, I remember my mother crying all the time and being depressed." She also recalls her mother suffering hunger and irritability. Holly's own case began with "depressions as far back as the beginning of high school. Severe, severe depression. It was like I couldn't find a solution for what was wrong at the time. I just wanted to die." It got worse when she started taking the pill at age nineteen. That's when she sought out a psychiatrist. "I have been in therapy for three or four years. Up until this point, I thought it might be psychological. That maybe I was mimicking my mother who was sick all those years." She always charted her mood swings and saw the menstrual connection, but still "doubted myself." She is clearly very grateful for the difference treatment has made: "Oh, my God. I have seen such a difference. I have been happy." The successful treatment also demonstrates to her that her complaints weren't symptoms of a psychodynamic problem with her mother.

We are also treating identical twins, Carla Mills and Sharon Cartwright, who were separated as children and given up for adoption. They have similar cases of PMS, marked by depression, anger, outbursts; both attribute their divorces to PMS. Carla was divorced once; Sharon twice. After locating each other in adulthood, they eventually found their natural mother and discussed PMS with her. Their mother and maternal grandmother had similar symptoms: depression, tension, headaches. Their mother said that she never felt well unless she was pregnant. Sharon remembers her mother as "always pregnant."

Many of our patients who have daughters, especially those in or approaching their teens, are fearful that the girls will develop premenstrual syndrome. Brenda Morgan has six children, including three daughters. "I'm watching them very closely because I just want to see that they are protected from this," she says. "If my daughters do develop it, there's no reason that they have to spend the major portion of their lives like I did, suffering. I spent most of my life thinking that I was probably insane and that I would wind up in an asylum sooner or later. That's an awful way to live. I hope the next generation would be spared this because of the growing understanding of PMS."

That view is echoed by Lauren Holloway, who has three children, including two girls, and whose mother also had premenstrual syndrome. Mrs. Holloway's condition grew from irritability and headaches that began when she started taking the birth control pill to extreme postpartum depression. "I think a lot about my own two daughters [and PMS]; this treatment is so wonderful that I want to go up on top of a mountain and shout to the world about it and help other women. I never understood what my mother's problem was when we were growing up," she says. "Mother was constantly going through different things. I've talked to my father about it. They divorced after thirty-six years of marriage. He just couldn't tolerate it anymore. We'd talk about what happened to her, and how she had her cravings and would go from doctor to doctor looking for an answer. They never found an answer but they always sent her home with something. That's the same thing they did with me. I found myself falling into the same pit. When I started crying and getting emotional and saying 'what is wrong with me?' my husband would call me Charlotte — that's my mother's name."

The disorder, like many genetic conditions, may skip a generation or two. Valerie Lawrence says her sisters and grandmothers have it, but her mother doesn't. Both grandmothers had multiple miscarriages and were treated with progesterone to help them carry a fetus to term. One of her sisters has "a peculiar case:" a life-threatening allergy to extreme changes of temperature, but only premenstrually. "If she's really hot and dives into a cool swimming pool or has been in the snow and is cold and comes in to sit by a fire, she'll 'blow up,' " Mrs. Lawrence says. "Her whole body turns red and she gets white welts — hives — all over and they itch like crazy. Twice she's been rushed to the hospital with her eyes, nose, and throat swollen shut; once her heart stopped."

Complications of Menstrual Synchrony

When both mother and daughter must face up to PMS each month, the tension in a household crackles, like an electric appliance threatening to short-circuit. Menstrual synchrony, a phenomenon as common as snow in Minnesota, usually plays a role in drawing the battle lines; women who live together or work together or spend inordinate amounts of time together often undergo subtle shifts in the timing of their menstrual cycles until all members of the circle experience the flow simultaneously. The pattern once was attributed to lunar phases, along with epileptic seizures and the birthing of babies. Whatever the cause, mutual cycles are a source of minor annoyance to some, especially to college students sharing bathrooms and tampon-dispensing machines, and a catalyst for violence in others. Some of our mother/daughter patients say they have come to blows over seemingly innocuous issues during a shared premenstrual phase. It's a potent situation when two women are locked in confrontation; it's near chaos when three or more women with PMS must negotiate turf and temper in the same home, the same office, the same locker room. When we interview patients, a frequent response to our questions about mood swings and other PMS behavior is "it's hard to figure out where my mother's symptoms left off and mine started."

Janice Feniman's story is a case in point. Her late mother had a severe case of premenstrual syndrome marked by tumultuous, violent behavior and drinking; her sisters also are burdened by it. "All of my sisters have mood swings. My oldest sister is on her third marriage and I think PMS was the cause of her divorces; she's also had a kind of hit or miss career life and that's because of her moods and depressions and outbursts. Our mother had a severe case. But I know that our maternal grandmother probably did not have it.

"My mother had difficulty with pregnancy and childbearing. Unfortunately she didn't know or care about birth control so she had five children and about four additional miscarriages and didn't enjoy being a mother," she recalls. "As I look back on it now, I am sure she had PMS because she was alternately a monster and a quiet, confused woman who just sort of muddled through life. She was not physically abusive to us, the children, thank heaven, but she was verbally abusive. She and my father were physically violent toward each other.

"I looked a lot like her and personality-wise I seemed like her. I was rather sensitive, easily hurt. So everyone said I was like my mother. That used to concern me a great deal. I just decided that I was going to survive. She apparently saw me as a threat to her; she always denied the good things that happened to me. There was nothing I could do to please her." After enduring for fifteen years one of the most complex cases of premenstrual syndrome that we have seen, Feniman was properly diagnosed and began progesterone therapy.

For many mothers and daughters, or sisters, or other women in close relationships with each other, the diagnosis is merely the starting point of a much more difficult stage: renegotiating the relationship. The women we treat frequently realize that their stormy travails with mothers or sisters were not due only to their premenstrual disorder, but were compounded by the other woman's case of PMS. They may have fueled a hostility to their mother over the years because of her outbursts and inexplicable reigns of terror over the family, labeling her a "witch" or worse. Erratic behavior and tantrums that seemed so vicious, unfair, and unloving to a child or adolescent are reinterpreted in light of the PMS pattern; now the daughter sees the mother as having suffered from an illness, and she's willing — sometimes eager — to accord the illness a sympathetic heart. Reconciliation is hardly simple, however. Mere mortals can't simply erase emotional damage inflicted over many years and redub the audio; there's a lot of static and garbling that has to be dealt with first. In most of these situations the women may need a third party to walk them through the initial awkward phase of establishing communication and pouring oil on still-turbulent waters. Counseling or psychotherapy can make the process easier for many.

Janice Feniman is one daughter who successfully bridged the gap with her mother. Once she began progesterone treatment at the clinic, she visited her mother and told her that she thought she had suffered from the condition all her life, that this hydra-headed disorder was the catalyst for the violence, the drinking, the temper tantrums. "We had a reconciliation of sorts; it wasn't easy. She didn't accept it at first," Feniman says. "But I just told her that knowing that her pain was like my pain made it okay; it just wiped the slate clean. She died last year but we had one full year of being a mother and daughter who came close to understanding each other."

SECTION III / *Living With PMS*

Chapter 9

*"All happy families are like one another;
each unhappy family is unhappy in its
own way."*

Leo Tolstoy, **Anna Karenina**

Strains on Relationships

"PMS is the woman's physiological problem but it is also a family problem. The family is tortured just as surely and constantly as the woman," commented one of our patients, a thirty-seven-year-old mother of four. Premenstrual syndrome is not just a painful and debilitating illness; its pattern of pendulum-like swings of mood and unpredictability burdens personal relationships and family life with an emotional load that would hobble a team of Clydesdales. The syndrome has been implicated in a host of family-oriented problems, from general discord to separation, divorce, and child abuse. The stormy personal relations in turn produce guilt and shame in the victim, a loss of self-esteem, and sense of being "bad." Ultimately women may become profoundly depressed and even suicidal.

In a PMS relationship, the husband of one of our patients says, "Your vulnerability has been violated. You learn that it's not really safe to be vulnerable to her because when she's in pain she'll use it against you. After several good days, though, you begin to be freer and open up, only to find that the cycle will begin again and you're vulnerable to her again. I remember going for days without saying anything — that's PMS baggage."

The slide from mild symptoms to the extreme can happen slowly, over a decade or more in some women, in a matter of months in others. It is difficult to halt the progressive decline and downward spiral. PMS women can't control their feelings or pain once the symptoms start, a moment our patients variously describe as a black cloud descending over them, an alien being seizing their body, an incubus that possesses them.

Single women often say that they limit their social life, particularly dating and intimacy with men, to the days of the month they are symptom-free. One management consultant told us that in the four years before she found treatment for her condition she saw two serious relationships disintegrate because the men couldn't understand why she wouldn't see them more than two weeks a month. One of them told her that he wanted more than an affair, he wanted a commitment. She was so confused and guilt-ridden by her PMS behavior that she didn't explain to him why she couldn't spend more time with him.

Another of our patients had managed to hide her problem from the man she dated for two years by making excuses, being unavailable, "out-of-town," or overworked during the five days each month that she felt unstable. During that time she refused to accept the fact that her condition was related to menstruation; rather she thought it was psychological and would go away. Eventually this couple married, and her husband became exposed to PMS for the first time. He told us that he thought at first that her outbursts and irritability were just part of the normal adaptation to married life, that she was finding the change from a single to a shared lifestyle stressful. As her physical complaints worsened, the strain on the marriage came close to tearing it apart. Compounding her physical problems was the guilt she felt over not disclosing her illness before the marriage. She ultimately sought treatment and saved her health and her relationship.

The most damaging symptoms to a relationship are irritability, anger, verbal and physical assaults, impulsiveness, loss of trust, suspicion or paranoia. Initially when the symptoms are mild and brief, the relationship returns to normal once they disappear. As the condition worsens and the cranky spouse becomes a raging tergament, the effect is disastrous. Gradually the man grows less tolerant and begins to react. Most men echo the voice of one husband who told us: "You don't know what's going on, yet you have a feeling that it's a biological thing. But you can't say anything or else she will accuse you of being a male chauvinist. But eventually you begin to strike back and say things you don't mean. Then she reacts to your anger and the relationship changes."

Guilt builds rapidly and continuously under this stress. During their symptom-free times, these women don emotional hair-shirts in their desperate efforts to rid themselves of a shrewish image and to compensate for the trouble they stirred up premenstrually. Apologies mount. Anticipation of the next cycle of symptoms fills their good days; they start to compress their life into the healthy period. They tell us that's when they cook, clean, spend time with their husband and children, and attend parties. Lydia Aarons, mother of two, lived with premenstrual syndrome for ten years. During the two years before she was properly treated, she was bedridden with blinding migraine headaches and depression. Aarons remembers those times vividly: "Sometimes we'd be with people and the women were all talking about little daily things, like wondering when they should change their baby's clothes from spring to summer weight, and I would be thinking about how I could cook twenty dinners by Friday. My reality was so much harsher than theirs. I had to do all my housework and cooking and everything during the one week I could function or else my husband or family would have to do it."

That pressure to do it all, even if they only have one week or two weeks a month in which they can fulfill their obligations, produces a great internal stress. Combined with the bewilderment the women feel over the source of their strife, their self-image starts to crumble like the facade of a building throttled by earth tremors. They think, "I should be able to control myself." They grit their teeth and say, "This month it will not happen." Their husband may say it. Their friends may say it. The next month, when the inevitable strikes, they feel violated, their will thwarted. After a few months, their self-esteem is destroyed. It's the natural reaction of any individual who has set herself — or himself, this is not a feminine phenomenon — up for repeated failure. When the sense of self worth is shaken, coping becomes a Sisyphean task; productivity and efficiency vanish. At this stage, depression descends.

Some men view their wife's freshly developed lack of self-esteem as an enemy that must be routed from the relationship. These men say they've lost respect for their mates, and they attack them verbally for giving up, for having grown unconfident, uncertain, indecisive. Premenstrual sufferers who can't cope with normal life can't cope with this flanking maneuver either; the result is always even more dissonance in the relationship, bringing it a few steps closer to destruction.

These are formidable obstacles to overcome for any couple. But as Karl Berman, a husband whose wife suffered with PMS for fifteen years, observes: "A PMS marriage that has endured is going to be a good marriage. Because if there are cracks and flaws in it to start with, it'll fall apart. Once they've found out what PMS is, they've had to weather some of the most hostile stress imaginable. Once you've handled a bad case of PMS, you can handle anything."

Husbands and Wives

The stories told by the couples who have lived with PMS are poignant and revealing. We've spent thousands of hours listening to their experiences; while the patterns are similar, the details are not.

Karen and Dan Shelton were high school and college sweethearts in Salt Lake City, the arid Western settlement founded by the followers of Joseph Smith, known as "Happy Valley" to the Mormon families who live in sight of the rose- and lavender-veined mountains. Married for sixteen years, they have five children. Karen Shelton recalls being distraught at one point in their courtship because "Dan had very seriously considered not marrying me because of my moodiness. I do remember being scared then. At the time I chalked up that part of me to coming from a verbally and sometimes physically abusive family." But they talked about it and decided to go ahead with the wedding.

Dan: "I always had a suspicion that there was something wrong. It's like buying a car. You drive it home and find a problem. You either make a decision to trade it in or have it repaired. I never liked it [the PMS episodes] but I thought, 'okay I will do what I have to do to make the marriage work, to make the car run again.' If good times weren't there, they would eventually return, a window of warmth was always there. There was an indication that there was something organically wrong. At worst, it could have been a form of mental illness. When she first found out about it being a hormonal thing, I felt a tremendous sense of relief that suspended judgment, that she wasn't to blame for this thing. That was a tremendous help. It was no fun. It's as horrible an experience for me now as it was then. Once you discover the cause of it, there's a target for your anger other than the person. Recognizing that kind of directed my anger. That discovery is a psychological release and relief. It doesn't do a great deal for the times you're caught up in it. I've given her a hard time about it. I've told her she's a hypochondriac. Lots of times when she says she can't help it, in the back of my mind I'd say 'sure, straighten up and fly right; control it.' Even now, when she flies off the handle, it's still difficult to deal with."

Communications are strong in the Shelton household, a factor that both say helped preserve their marriage.

Dan: "We're a very verbal couple. We don't hold a lot inside. I'm sure a lot of fears I had we were able to talk about and work out. Recognizing PMS doesn't make it any easier for the victim or the family. You still feel horrible. You still have trouble handling it." After one violent argument the two had, he told Karen, 'You're so good when you're good. You're so wonderful when you're well.'

Karen: "When I'm having an outburst, most human beings would have taken a swipe at me. But not Dan." He is, in fact, "usually non-combative. That was aggravating to me."

Dan: "If I'd hit her every time I had thought about it, she wouldn't be here now... I recognized that there were times when something would seem to burst inside her and she would come apart. She always felt so sorry afterward. She'd always apologize and she was so rational then. One of the aspects of my character is that I'm very forgiving. I'm incapable of carrying a grudge very long. In fact, I don't carry grudges. That's been a real blessing. If we hadn't been able to get beyond that, we'd be carrying around some pretty heavy baggage that could only be destructive to our relationship."

Identifying the Pattern

Many mates of women with PMS observed the relationship between the outbursts and health problems and the menstrual cycle long before the women themselves.

Richard Paton kept a diary of the behavior and outbursts of his wife, Ann, for three years before she was diagnosed as a PMS victim; he had been aware of their cyclical occurrence for many years before that. "I became aware that her angry and depressed times were related to her periods about nine years ago," he says. "Every time we'd have a fight I'd go running upstairs and look at her package of birth control pills. There were always two or three pink ones left. I came to recognize that when there were two or three left, it was family battle time again. I was very aware of a group of signs that said 'Here it comes again.' Sometimes I could see her going like a whirlwind, cleaning the house, generally at absurd times of the day, and I knew that it was coming."

Ann says of her husband: "He caught on to PMS before I did." Once she caught him marking the calendar for the new year on the days that he thought would be one week before her period. "I got very angry. I thought it was sneaky, notetaking behind my back. He wouldn't bring it up in conversation, and when I tried to bring it up, he wouldn't be interested. But he saw the pattern, and he saw an enormous change in me the first month that I took the progesterone."

Why did Richard track her cycles? "I don't like to fight. I don't receive well. I get angry and lash out as much as she does, which, of course, makes the arguments worse. Keeping track helped me to modify my reactions. I knew I had to treat her very lightly and very warily during those times. The most terrible times between us always happened then."

Timing was also important because he travels regularly on business and tried to arrange to stay home when he knew that she was premenstrual. "I didn't think that the kids needed it. She had to lash out and it was better me than them. Sometimes I wanted to be away during the worst two or three days. Then she'd use the phone instead of the kids. I'd be in a hotel room somewhere, and I'd put the phone down on the bed and go to the bathroom or read a book. She wouldn't even notice. It was that type of haranguing."

Ann says, "Almost always, the fights would be over my criticism of his behavior. I could hear myself, a crazy woman saying 'I know you didn't go down to the village to buy stamps, you went down to call someone.' [He had an affair once, during her first pregnancy.] I'd be very suspicious and paranoid. I felt as if everyone were out to get me, especially him. I couldn't count on him and I couldn't trust him. No one could help me."

Her irrationality was confined to the two-week period before she began to menstruate. "I had control over myself during those other two weeks. When I'd have a crazy thought then I'd dismiss it. During the two weeks before my period, I'd obsess over it. The same crazy thought, over and over, like a broken record." When she behaved irrationally, "My husband would say 'Oh, Christ, here we go again,' and slam the door and leave, or sometimes he'd turn on me. We're still married and I love him very much. We have a good marriage. When something's going on, I try to remember how awful I must have been to live with then."

Her relationship with her husband became "extremely tenuous." During her premenstrual time, "If I didn't get too aggressive and I let him know that I needed him, everything would be all right. But if I turned my depression and anxiety into an attack, he'd back off. I used to feel that I was at his mercy, that he made a conscious decision to help me or not — now I see that it probably depended on how hostile I was. Sometimes I'd be able to see quite lucidly that the whole problem was mine, and that he was doing the best that he could. Other times, I'd blame how I was feeling on him.''

Distance didn't stem the outbursts, Richard says: "Sometimes during a trip I'd sit in my hotel room fuming with anger: not reading, not watching television. Just angry. Every month she'd accuse me of being unfaithful. 'You're a bastard, look what you did to me.' And I'd think, 'God, won't she ever forget. Won't she ever stop bringing this up?' ''

They frequently battled over the telephone. "One night I was in a hotel in Cincinnati, and she called and we began to argue. I hung up, and she called back. I hung up on her again and called the hotel desk to tell them not to put any more calls through. 'Not even calls from my office or from my wife.' '' When she called for the third time, the hotel operator wouldn't put her call through. When Ann threatened to call the hotel management and the police, the operator called Richard and told him *she'd* call the police. So he called his wife and said, "The cops will come to our house, too, and take you to the funny farm." After hours of talking, he said, she finally hung up.

He reacted very strongly to their fights. "The depression that I felt, I think I was as low as anyone could get. He realized that her problems were physical and cyclical, but "I was terrified of breaking up our marriage and destroying our beautiful family." Richard said that to outsiders, "We were the happiest couple alive." Some of their friends were aware that they had marital problems, but "it didn't seem relevant to tell people that it was cyclical." Their marriage counselor, also a good friend, once told him, "I don't understand how you two can be at each other's throats and still be a perfect host and hostess for eight people at dinner. We told each other that, even with everything, we probably had a better marriage than most people. Our lives were only difficult twenty-five percent of the time. But in the last three years, the stress period stretched to about two weeks of the month."

Progesterone therapy has eliminated her symptoms, changing their lives considerably. "If I had known what the cause was and that someone in the world was working on it, well, I would have been thrilled. Now I say 'This is the PMS reacting.' I try to be understanding. If she yells, I'm still angry, but later I tell myself that it's just the PMS." Since she began treatment, "There's happiness in our family now."

And Ann says she deals with her husband much differently now that the progesterone permits her to control her reactions. "I realized that I can walk away from a potential fight by stating how I feel about the situation and being solution-oriented, instead of flipping out and getting irrational."

Martin Schanberg, like Richard Paton, also saw the pattern of PMS long before his wife, Felicia, did. Her sharp mood swings and outbursts had led the couple to two gynecologists and four psychiatrists before she was properly diagnosed. The second psychiatrist wanted to put her in a psychiatric hospital. "I thought there was something wrong with my brain," she recalls. But Martin Schanberg suggested that her moods were caused by a chemical imbalance. He told her that he could "feel" her cycles. She got angry and said, "It has nothing to do with my period. It's just something the matter with me." Her husband told all the psychiatrists, "She's not like this all the time, just before her period." But, she says, the doctors, "shrugged it off." Her symptoms became aggravated after the birth of their first child. "I noticed that she would get like that at the same time each month, about a week or two before her period. As time went on, I realized that it had to be physical."

He said he'd lie awake in bed and try to analyze the problem. "I'd ask myself how I could be such a terrible person. I don't drink or play around, and I'm home, helping around the house a lot. I didn't know how I could be hurting her so much." Martin found dealing with her during her premenstrual time disheartening and frustrating. "Nothing I said was right. I couldn't help her."

"During my bad times, I would be angry and irritable," Felicia says. "And very clumsy. I would drop things and burn dinners. My husband used to say, 'You know dinner's ready when the smoke alarm goes off.' I'd burn toast and eggs all the time." Those jokes of Martin infuriated her because she couldn't seem to stop the episodes. "I kept ruining things and dropping things and breaking things because my mind was somewhere else."

The Schanbergs have an extensive collection of anecdotes about Felicia's lack of coordination. Martin recalls a Father's Day a few years ago when the family decided to go for a drive. "She wanted to take our second car, because our boat and trailer were hooked up to the station wagon. We have a sloping driveway: you can't see the bottom of the driveway from the garage. I stood on the lawn and watched her back the car into the station wagon and the boat." He found it depressing at the time, but now he thinks the incidents are funny.

Martin: "I used to tell our friends that my wife had her priorities mixed up: she'd add too much water to the washing machine and too little to the potatoes. She was always burning vegetables." He says that he used to get upset but after a while he got used to it. "I saw how hard she tried to avoid accidents. She just couldn't help it. The clumsiness was part of the pattern. Two weeks she'd be fine and the other two she'd be awful. She'd trip over things. She sliced an onion for a salad one day and almost sliced off her finger." One day she smashed a glass on the counter, cut her hand, and watched the blood drip onto the floor. "I knew it was time to go to my room until it all passed."

Sometimes her absentmindedness approached dangerous levels. On her husband's birthday Felicia made his favorite cake. After she put the cake into the oven, she saw a can of Raid on the counter and realized that she had sprayed the pans with insecticide instead of with Pam, the aerosol vegetable oil. As she threw the cake batter out, a friend walked in. "Where are you going?" he asked. "I'm going to the store to buy more eggs," she said. "I have to make another cake because I used Raid instead of Pam on the pans." He laughed, she said, but she didn't find it particularly funny.

When she was diagnosed in our office, she felt exuberant. "Maybe I'll finally have a good Thanksgiving and Christmas." On progesterone therapy, her symptoms have completely disappeared. The difference, Martin says, is all internal. "No one knew what was going on. From the outside we're a model family, our friends and neighbors are probably envious of us." She has not convinced her family doctor or her sister, who is a nurse, that PMS was the cause of her problems. Her family doctor said, "It's rubbish. They've brainwashed you." The other people she talks to are also skeptical but, she says, "I know it's real."

Social Tensions

Unpredictable, unpleasant, sometimes vicious or argumentative, women in the midst of the premenstrual torment are usually not capable of dealing with polite society. Stung by their penchant for verbal darts and gibes at the most inappropriate moments, friends and relatives grow alienated, spouses withdraw or refuse to accompany their mates anywhere that they think they might act out.

Kevin Larson, whose wife Marla had PMS for seventeen years, says: "I can't count the number of times we were invited to go places, when I'd say 'I'm not going with you anyplace like this.' We'd bow out. You begin to manufacture excuses very effectively. One woman at a PMS support group meeting said she used to tell people she had epilepsy so she could get out of social things without completely losing her friends. Marla would talk about her horrible back problems — which she really has — or that she was so tired or run down since the baby was born — which she was — or that her thyroid was acting up — which it was. They were legitimate bases for excuses but they were crutches for the real reason. That would precipitate a lot of guilt feelings. But it got to the point where it just didn't bother me anymore that we never went anywhere."

One husband terms his social adaptation to PMS "self-preservation maneuvers." He says, "You've got to drag your wife around when she doesn't feel good. At parties, you fill in, or you abandon her. I would find myself talking with people, having a great time, and Janet would be sitting across the room in a corner by herself or stuck talking to someone whom she couldn't cope with but couldn't seem to discourage from sitting with her. She'd say, 'Please don't ever leave me by myself at a party.' She couldn't handle it. You begin to think that your wife is damaged goods, that she's got a problem. So you accept it and say 'if that's what's got to be done, okay.' But it wasn't okay, and you knew that, you resented that."

Social strains lead many couples "to become kind of reclusive," according to another husband, Mark Halloran. "I'm not a real gregarious person, I don't have a lot of close friends. If people came over, it was kind of a hassle. It wasn't fun. Judy would plan things when she was feeling well — birthday parties, dinner parties. Then the day would come and she'd feel lousy."

Judy Halloran remembers: "When I'd plan them, I'd be fine. Then ten days later, I'd inevitably feel terrible. There I was, trapped by a decision I'd made. Women who have PMS tend not to know it or not to realize that every month the symptoms hit. They have convenient amnesia for the kind of suffering they go through each month and so when they're feeling well, they plan things as though they were always well."

Locked in a body they no longer understand, caught up in deeds and spewing out words they instantly regret, the women themselves soon have no interest in anything but coping with the syndrome. A common feeling, expressed by hundreds of women, is a dread of social get-togethers and parties during the premenstrual time. One of our patients, Roberta Carl, says, "Sometimes I felt as if I were a nebulous blob. I sat there mute. I couldn't talk or be social."

Ingrid Low, a forty-five-year-old mother of six, recalls: "My whole life used to be planned about what was going to happen those two weeks before my period. I couldn't go any place, I couldn't make any plans, I would literally crawl into a shell, or have to hide in my bedroom for four to five days. This is no longer the case; progesterone has really changed everything. I couldn't take stress at all in that period of time. I couldn't handle a holiday or a birthday; it would just be a total knockout time for me. It's an amazing, almost indescribable difference, considering that I'm forty-five and I've lived with this since I've been a teenager. I'm lit-erally a new person (after being on progesterone therapy.). My husband and I have been married for twenty-five years and I think this is the first one year the man has ever had. The difference is unbelievable."

The Last Phase: Divorce

Over time, premenstrual syndrome drives a wedge between husband and wife that leads them to discuss or threaten divorce; for many it actually leads to the courtroom. About twenty to twenty-five percent of our patients have been divorced; five to ten percent of the total have been divorced more than once. All of these women cite PMS as the primary cause of the split; the former spouses we've talked to confirm this. Most women we've treated have managed to save their marriages, but the damage done by their illness has left permanent scars.

Cynthia and Larry Wilson played out the same scenario hundreds of times. "Her bags would be packed, and she'd walk out the back door to the garage to leave," Larry says. "I'd race out the front door to catch her. I'd pick her up and carry her back inside. We'd fall on the kitchen floor and I'd hold onto her." When she felt better, she'd apologize. She would tell him that she didn't know how he could stand her, and asked him why he didn't leave. "Because I love you," he told her. "You know that in two weeks you'll be happy and enjoying things again." But when she was premenstrual, he couldn't reach her.

Sally Ziegler, a nurse and mother of two, says of her disintegrating relationship with her husband, Joe: "Nothing he ever did or said to me was right when I was having my symptoms. When he was sweet and dear, I'd tell him he was patronizing and condescending. If he were angry or hostile, I said he was a son of a bitch and he didn't care and he wasn't good to me. If he tried to ignore me, I said he was too passive, which he wasn't. There was no behavior he could adopt that was right with me. I gave him an impossibly hard time. I did tell him he ought to leave me, that we should get a divorce. I'd say, 'if you can't take it, go. I can't bear the guilt.' We sat down and talked about it. I was crying and hysterical. He felt angry toward me. He's a very reserved, introverted, very proper, very closed type of person. Once he threw a plate on the floor in frustration over me. There was always a part of me that was still there, buried deep inside." Now Joe and Sally are going to a marriage counselor.

Another of the many couples who have stitched their marriage together with the help of marriage counseling or therapy is Lisa and Mike Ritter. Mike Ritter says that even during his wife's tirades, their two boys remained their priority. "If she asked me for a divorce, I'd say 'Okay, but I'm not leaving.' I'd tell her that she had to be the one to leave." Only once, he said, did he leave. He stayed with friends for a week to "cool off." Sometimes she'd say, "I'll move out because you're a better father than I am a mother. The boys will be better off with you." Then he said, "It would all blow over and we'd be there cuddling."

Another husband, Steve Hart says: "When Laura would offer to give me a divorce, of course I'd sometimes think 'You bet, let's do it.' But then I'd stop and think. We made a very strong commitment by getting married. But she's not offering a divorce to me, really. She's hitting herself over the head with guilt, just punishing herself for her bad behavior. You see through that very quickly. No. Why would I ever leave her? I love her. Love is more than just a passion. Love is a commitment. That's what holds it together. It's rock-hard cement. It's a commitment that lasts long after the passion has cooled down. That's love. Come hell or high water. I think after saying I love her for ten or twelve years, it's not a lie on my part. I do care about her. I do love her.''

For some, love is not strong enough mortar to fuse the fragments of the marriage together. The specter of the syndrome becomes too great a weight for the marriage to bear and divorce is inevitable.

Ariana Buren, a schoolteacher with three children, has been divorced twice. ''My husbands found it difficult to cope with me, the second one especially. It's a different situation. My children are from my first marriage. I was very much in love with my second husband, and still am. We had a lot of extraneous problems. We lived together before we were married, we both had children from prior marriages. It was very difficult. He was aware that something was going on with me that was cyclical. If I were premenstrual, I would drink a lot and become very argumentative and hysterically depressed. Certainly that was not an easy thing to cope with.''

Despite her return to health, she is still sorting out the emotional problems from her recent divorce and move into a new apartment and new job. ''It's a very different type of feeling that I have now. It's just all those things I have to cope with, and trying to get them straightened out.''

Catherine Rodriguez, thirty-two, a government lawyer and mother of a five-year old boy, also has been divorced twice. Her first divorce in 1970 ''may have been related to PMS.'' But her second divorce in 1980 after a two-year separation she feels was definitely attributable to PMS. ''I was an absolutely royal, unhappy bitch.'' Each month she felt out of control, angry, and depressed. She would sleep all weekend. When she wasn't sleeping she would abuse her husband, verbally and physically [throwing dishes at him]. When she first heard of progesterone therapy for PMS, she thought ''it was too easy a way out,'' and couldn't believe that her depressions were organically caused. Now, she says, she feels ''born again.'' She thought that life was something to be endured; now it's ''something to be enjoyed.'' Last New Year's she got back together with her ex-husband who was ''disbelieving, but hopeful.'' Their relationship is now solid, but she has decided for other reasons not to re-marry him.

Coping with Success

Once diagnosed and under treatment for premenstrual syndrome, most of our patients report a disappearance of virtually all of their symptoms within one to three cycles. Some women, who have difficulty identifying the correct day on which to start the progesterone therapy, or absorb the progesterone poorly, or who have extreme cases of depression or migraine, may have one or two "bad" days for the first few months of treatment. But even these days, they say, are never as severe as their symptoms were when the PMS was untreated. The relief, surprise, and joy at having the yoke of premenstrual syndrome lifted is a heady emotional experience. But successful treatment creates its own share of problems for many families. Any dramatic change in the circumstances of a relationship, even a turn for the better, upsets the equilibrium of the situation. We encourage our patients to join local support groups for PMS families that have sprung up around the country, or to seek family therapy or counseling if they need a third party to help them rebuild their bridges to each other.

As Lindsey Leckie, director of the National PMS Society, based in Durham, N.C., explained: "Couples often have a lot of 'scarring' and guilt overlay. It's hard just to go out and have a good time. There's about a two-month interval after a woman sees improvement when she expects the most support. But for most couples, it seems to be the most trying time. A lot of the husband's pent-up hostility and anger over the illness surfaces, especially the stuff he didn't vent before because his wife was vulnerable." The organization she heads, which she co-founded with Patty Cannon, is the catalyst of a national network of support groups; at this writing sixty-five groups were active nationally, providing help for PMS families and dozens more are started each month. "I don't think attending support group meetings is a lifelong thing. Some people cycle in and cycle out quite quickly. They're able to work through the problem they've got and then they get out of it. We want to offer temporary support. With less severe cases the need is of shorter duration. A lot of husbands and wives do stay for a long time, usually more severe cases of longer duration. The support group is an important way to reach out to the men in the lives of women with PMS. They need to forgive themselves for the anger they've felt and the guilt they feel. The husbands' reactions to meeting other men is amazing — instant relief, empathy."

One patient, a thirty-seven-year-old tax attorney in Atlanta, who is married and has a brood of eight children and stepchildren to raise, says, "PMS spreads out to the family. The family is not quick to forget. You go through your two weeks of pain and emotional depression. When you come out of it you feel so good that you expect them to say, 'Oh, she feels good now; that really wasn't her before.' But it doesn't work that way. The scars of the PMS time have to continuously be dealt with. Things were said during that period that you really didn't mean. Things were done during that period that you really didn't mean to do."

Cynthia Wilson says her children weren't as suspicious of her "cured" self as her husband Larry was. "In a romantic way and in a giving way, Larry had a hard time taking it. He was afraid that kind of giving would stop and the witch in me would come back. It hurt me that he wouldn't respond more overtly. I used to ask myself 'Has he stopped loving me?' We've had a lot of talks about it. Now when I reach out and everything's great, he'll accept it."

Dealing with the scars, the guilt, the painful memories and getting on to a new life is enormously difficult. The key, perhaps, is forgiveness. As Hannah Arendt wrote: "...no man can forgive himself and no one can be bound by a promise made only to himself... The possible redemption from the predicament of irreversibility — of being unable to undo what one has done — is the faculty of forgiving." Since one can't simply demand the forgiveness of the people who feel hurt, a women recovered from PMS needs to realize that understanding, patience, and time are her best tools in regaining her family's trust. Sometimes, of course, the wounds cut too deep to be bound by a Band-Aid. In these families, the best suggestion is to obtain psychological counseling.

In addition, the women newly rid of the syndrome finds that her family may have high expectations of her. Valerie Lawrence's experience was typical. "All of a sudden I'm okay, where once I was incapacitated three weeks out of every four. I've got two kids and a husband who's got great expectations. Unless I'm in bed with a migraine, I'm supposed to be wonder woman all the time. It's a sort of feeling that you've been Rip Van Winkle. It's very exciting and it's a great challenge. There's also an insecurity from a background of having not been well enough to do anything for ten years. Last year I had Christmas for the first time in a decade. I enjoyed it. But there are days when feeling good can also bring a daunting, overwhelming sense.

Don't misunderstand me, I feel wonderful and never, never would want to re-live the last ten years of my life.''

Overall, the sentiment of women who have defeated the PMS rage inside them, with lifestyle changes and progesterone therapy, say they know they're at a new frontier. As Susan Pearson, a magazine editor and mother of three who is one of the survivors, put it: ''Now's a time for healing, a time to explore new aspects of our relationship. It's still scary, but it's the most satisfying time of my whole marriage. I think we're lucky to be living now. All the other women with PMS lived and died without any help at all. We're pioneers.''

The Children

The innocent victims of PMS are the children of mothers with the disorder. Children are very aware of and sensitive to any changes in their mother's personality, behavior, and emotional reactions, and how that translates into her treatment of and responses to them. Younger children will tend to withdraw, thinking her outbursts and illness are because of something they've done. But older children, especially adolescent girls, are more likely to respond in kind. This is a pattern of reaction also seen in children of divorce, and in children whose parent or sibling is extremely ill or has died. When the security of their home is jeopardized, when they sense they can't count on the all-encompassing, all-forgiving warmth of mother, they grow uncertain, suspicious, or hostile.

One woman, a bookkeeper in Delaware who is divorced and has two children, says, ''My daughter took responsibility for my violent mood swings; she thought it was her fault. When I first found out that I wasn't crazy, that I had an illness, she said, 'Mom, it would be great if the doctor could help you, but what if your problem is caused by children?''' Not all children articulate their fears so directly, but most of them have similar feelings.

The mothers' views of their relationships with their children are a study in anger, verbal outbursts, occasional spankings that the women later regretted. In our experience the physical abuse of children is rare in women with PMS, except in the most extreme cases. Most women go to great lengths to avoid hitting or abusing their children; they'll leave the room, leave the house, send the child on an errand, anything that will put some distance between their children and their feelings of rage. Only one of our patients has ever said that her treatment of her children approached abuse. Monica Randolph, forty-six, is the mother of five children, three of whom are one year apart in age. When they were toddlers and she was also taking care of her mother's two youngest babies, she says "my kids were almost battered. I'm ashamed to say it, but it's probably true. I never wanted to lose my temper with them and god knows, I wouldn't have consciously abused them. But when I was taking care of five babies under the age of three at the same time and I would be in the premenstrual phase, I was like a keg of dynamite. I didn't know where these feelings of rage came from, but I couldn't control them. The oldest is twenty-six now and my kids don't seem to have any emotional scars. They spend a lot of time at home, we talk a lot, we have a good relationship. They know I would never intentionally hurt them. I love them more than I could ever say."

Many mothers develop enormous guilt over their failure to attend their children's music recitals, Little League baseball games, science fairs, and the like because of their condition. One mother's comment is an echo of hundreds we've heard: "On the day of my daughter's violin recital, I managed to drive her there, but I couldn't stay. Everyone else's mother was there, but I couldn't stay. My daughter didn't say anything to me, but I knew that she was disappointed. I felt so guilty."

Ronnie Albert still remembers how "I ruined my son's birthday outing." She and her husband were taking the boy to Broadway, to see the musical *Annie*. As they drove into Manhattan from their suburban home, she says, "I could feel that awful, heavy, painful feeling. I was so deadened with depression that I could hardly move. Fifteen minutes into the show, I went to the ladies room and stayed there, crying, during the entire performance."

The most universal experiences of these mothers are the day-to-day feelings of rage, the confrontations with their children.

Wilma Cohen: "I couldn't talk to my children. The physical feeling was that the inside of my body was going at one hundred miles an hour. If you could imagine that. Sometimes I couldn't cope with very minor things. If my husband walked through the door, I'd just announce that I was going to bed, 'take care of the kids.' I just had to walk away from everybody. Sometimes I would just storm out of the house, get into my car and drive, just to get that feeling out of my body. I felt like everyone at that time, my children especially, were suffering. I'd scream at them. I'd downgrade them. And you know, I consider myself a very good mother.''

The outbursts and anger, the complete unpredictability of their mothers, makes younger children withdraw emotionally and physically, while children old enough to play anywhere out of their mother's striking range leave the room or the house. Teenagers tend to spend as little time as possible around their mothers, although adolescent girls may rebel and fight back once a confrontation starts.

Joan Wagner, a thirty-two-year-old secretary, is married and the mother of two children: ''I would get up in the morning and scream at the kids because they tipped over a glass of milk. I tried to tell them what was happening, that my symptoms were physical, but I didn't really understand what was going on myself. My son would say, 'I can't stand you, Mother.' My husband didn't know what to do, so he'd say, 'Mom's sick now, so leave her alone.' ''

Repairing the damage that premenstrual syndrome inflicts on the relationship between mother and child is a long and emotionally painful process. Most mothers with PMS spend a considerable amount of time explaining and apologizing to their children about their problem, emphasizing that the outbursts and erratic episodes are not directed at the children and do not mean that their mothers do not love them.

Penny Rhodes has six children, ranging from twelve to twenty-three. ''The older ones, it really took a tremendous chunk out of their lives. They never knew how they'd find their mother. I'd be a lovely person for about two weeks, but when they came to the door they never knew what they were going to find. They don't seem to have any particular scars left on their life at this point that are very noticeable, but of course I've spent a lot of time talking to them and going through the whole process of explaining. They understand the illness and what caused it, so they've made very good adjustments. I would say in their younger years, they had a very difficult time. It basically colored their whole life at that point.''

Carolyn Grant had migraine headaches so severely that she would lie in a dark room for two to six days because the pain was so severe. Her husband helped with the children and housework. ''I have fantastic children. They were very responsible at a very early age. I'd get up in the morning and put cereal on the table, get them off to school, and go back to bed." Sometimes, she said, her children would bring her tea in bed. But, she said, the children noticed that she was different on certain days. She remembers that her younger son said to her, "Mommy, you're really confused. I told you that three times already."

Importance of Fathers' Role

Fathers can play a key role in helping the children cope with this stress in their lives.

Dan Shelton explains how he tried to help his children cope with their mother's illness: "Any husband will feel assaulted, feel hurt, and sometimes hurt irreparably. But he realizes he's got to do something and help out. Ultimately, he has to be responsible for the children. In some cases, the kids may be abused. They're helpless at home with her all day. It's very difficult for him to keep saying to the kids, 'let's just leave her here to stew in her own juices.' It's very hard for kids not to take it personally. I take it personally. You respond to it in a human way. Kids haven't developed to that point. They probably ask themselves, 'Why does this lady hate me?' What it requires is a lot of overcompensation. Mothers are usually the all-loving parent and father is the taskmaster, whose love is more conditional. With PMS, in our family, we tried to overcompensate but to be very consistent with them so the kids would feel secure. If Karen's having a tough time, I'll take the kids into a room and read them a story or talk to them about school in a matter-of-fact, light way, as if nothing unusual was going on. I'd just say, 'Mom's hormones are out of whack today so just stay away from her.' There's an element of survival here. If it was really bad, I'd say, 'Hey, Tom, get on your bike. Go into the garden. Go play with a friend. Don't say anything. Don't make any sounds.' The kids learn that if they cut up too much, Karen would explode. Any PMS relationship is tainted with caution. Tom talks about it off the cuff even."

Karen Shelton recalls the day her ten-year-old son asked, "How can I be sure I don't marry somebody with PMS?" It startled her, she says, but "I didn't take offense at it. I'm sure he didn't mean that he didn't love me. But I told him, jokingly, to take a menstrual calendar with him on his dates to have the girl fill it out. Our daughter is very quiet and doesn't talk about anything much or ask me about PMS, but she's at a stage where she gets into snits occasionally and gets sassy, runs into her room. Her brother teases her when she does that by telling her she has PMS. She just can't handle that. Tom told her she would definitely have it because I have it and it runs in families. She just gets very upset when he says that.''

Robert Quint says, "I'd tell the kids that we had to grin and bear it, not to argue with their mother because it was a difficult time for her.'' Generally, he said, the children never asked what was wrong. But sometimes their son would get frustrated when he couldn't understand why his mother was angry. Quint told him to put up with it, that there was nothing they could say or do that would please her when she felt like that. And he'd remind him how his mother was the other two weeks. She was a wonderful mother then, he said. But he adds, "If I tried to discipline the kids when she was premenstrual, she'd jump in to defend them and we'd have a fight. The kids would watch from the sidelines. During the other two weeks, when she was fine, I'd be afraid to go near them.''

With her symptoms under control, their family situation has improved dramatically. "The house is more carefree. My daughter doesn't hide in her room anymore, my son's grades have improved, and he's more involved in extracurricular activities at school.'' But, he says, the change is discernible only to the family. "No one knew what was going on. From the outside we're a model family. Our friends and neighbors are probably envious of us.''

Paul Clinton shepherded his two sons around the explosions of their mother's temper. "Most of the time,'' he says, "the boys knew when to step aside. They're good friends and the older boy is very understanding. They'd go off into their bedroom or the family room, and I'd shuttle between them, trying to help her and telling them 'Mommy has a headache, just sit quietly and play.' Our older boy, who's ten, is a very enigmatic child. He just closed off his feelings. He'd play Dad with his younger brother. I heard him say, 'That's just Mom and Dad going at it again.' ''

Clinton remembers some "nasty scenes'' when they were threatening each other with divorce and the children would be in bed with them. The younger one would cry and say, "Don't do it." The older one wouldn't say anything. The older boy would comfort the younger boy. The early stages of their fights often were in front of the kids. Clinton adds, "How we have such super kids, I don't know." Two or three times, he took the children out to dinner to get them away from her. "But when we had our worst fights, her source of comfort would be the kids, and she'd take them out." He noticed that she took them to the zoo three times "to curry favor."

Initially he didn't want to discuss PMS with the boys. "I didn't want to set them up against their mother. But they've watched plenty of fights." According to him, she never threw anything at him in front of the children, "but they would hear the crash... Kids mature faster in this type of atmosphere. I finally explained to him (the oldest) that women get a period and that all women react differently. Some get cramps, some get grouchy. Mommy doesn't hate me as much as she seems to, it's just that time of month." He feels that the ten-year-old understood, but the seven-year-old didn't. The older child would say to him, "I understand Dad," but he didn't respond past that. "It's probably part of the loyalty thing that children have toward their parents," Clinton says.

Clinton knows the marital strife and PMS "has affected the boys to a certain extent. Children react when they watch their parents fighting and yelling at each other. They'd come down and see glass on the floor and hear me calling their mother drunken and crazy. There have to be scars. Now, though, "I feel they're very secure. I'm sure our youngest thinks of the past sometimes, but he's content. Sean, who's ten, is going through a stage. He's sure of those who love him; he's less sure of himself." He thinks the affection that he and Joanna show each other is the best thing for their children. "We're very demonstrative. We'd be hugging and kissing and working together in the kitchen when things were good. It was part of a reassurance program."

He says that now his son is older, he talks more, but he never brings up the past. He remembers once driving with him and saying, "You realize that things are much better in the house now that Mom has been treated." His son said, "Yes, I know. That's why she's in Boston [at our center] today."

Another couple also says their children adapted without much apparent difficulty to their disrupted home. But their mother makes a concerted effort to explain her illness to them and otherwise compensate if she's treated them unfairly. "I apologize to the kids if I'm having a PMS day," she says. Her husband adds, "I don't think there's any indication that they love her any less because she has PMS. They don't like PMS. They respond in their own way to it. Families recall incidents involving mothers and children that range from terrific battles to loving scenes of understanding.

Doug Richards, the eleven-year-old son of Martha Richards, relates an incident when his mother's anger cascaded over the household seemingly without reason. Doug had been playing outside in the yard. "Mom called me and I went into the house. She grabbed me and said, 'where've you been? I called you fifty times.' She chased me around the house with a flyswatter. Then she pushed me on the couch and hit me and said, 'Don't you ever do that again.' While she was chasing me around, the dinner burned. She threw all the food on the floor and when Dad came in there was food all over the kitchen. Sometimes I thought she was crazy. She'd yell and scream for no reason. But she was fine when she wasn't getting her period." Generally, he'd try to avoid her. His father would tell him, "Mom's in a bad mood, so don't upset her," and he'd stay in his room.

Claire Pettit tells of the night "when I had just put the baby to bed and my husband was giving our daughter, who was four, a bath. I had told my daughter about my problem and my cycle and everything. The two of them were laughing and playing in the bath. I just blew up at the noise and really fussed at them. I said if they woke up the baby they'd have to take care of him. At that, I saw my husband bend over to console Jennifer after my outburst. She just reached up and patted him on the leg and said, 'It's okay, Daddy. It's just her time of month.' "

When Ruth Watson, a thirty-five-year-old mother of two, explained to her son that "two weeks before I get my period, my body changes and I feel sad," he said, "Mommy, I wish I could help you." The children really notice the difference in her behavior now that she's been treated. "One day when I was getting nervous and irritable, my son said, 'Maybe you should take your medicine.' And it was past the time that I should have taken it."

Some parents, especially the mothers, say they find it hard not to overcompensate with their children for the pain they've introduced into their lives. For most PMS families, as with divorced couples, this may take the form of granting the children special privileges, easing up on normal discipline, taking them on special trips, to restaurants, or spending larger-than-normal sums of money on toys, games, and clothes. Cathy Berman, who has coped very well with her family in general, admits that her two children lack very little. "I have to admit to some kind of overindulgence with the kids because of the situation we have. I've been overindulging in clothing departments. They can have anything they want in clothes. I feel that I'm trying to compensate a lot for the outbursts and tension in the house. My mother [who also had PMS] did that. We were rather spoiled materially. There wasn't a lot we didn't have in the material sense. Christmas was a very elaborate time. The toy store would be in our living room on Christmas morning."

Advice to Husbands From the Spouse of a PMS Victim

At a seminar on PMS last year, the husband of a woman who has suffered from the disorder for fifteen years addressed a standing-room-only crowd that included more than one hundred husbands. He focused his attention on their concerns, telling them:

"Let me tell you what your life is like. The line between love and hate is very thin. You have accused your wife, your sweetheart, of hypochondria. You have unpaid medical bills sitting on the desk. You are tired of sending her in for tests because they don't work, they don't show anything. You're tired of her being on Valium, or tired of her being on painkillers. You're tired of doing the babysitting because there are times when she'll lock herself in her room. You're tired of getting the kids off to school in the morning because she can't get out of bed. Your social life is shot because you find that when you go to parties you can't stay very long sometimes during the difficult periods.

"You find that there are long periods of silence. You find that there are arguments at home. You find harsh words, you find fights. You find every now and again secret stores of chocolate; you find Coca-Cola in the refrigerator; you find little caches of food. These women are crazy for sweets or caffeine because it helps them.

"You suffer in silence. You discover that there may indeed be some violence, not intended, but spontaneous. Maybe you find paint peeling around the door frame where the door has been slammed so many times that the paint is falling off. Perhaps you find that your wife can't stand noise, she can't stand to watch the football game, she can't stand to see those things on TV that are violent and stressful because that upsets her. You've discovered that she doesn't exercise because exercise is painful. You discover her helplessness, and you find yourself being helpless alternately with being resolute and courageous and saying, 'I can cope with this.' And then alternately saying to yourself, 'I can't deal with this one more day, one more hour.' You find yourself mutually discussing divorce, thinking about it, or perhaps going even further and actually going through with it. I've talked to lots of husbands and they universally feel these things. And you don't know what's going to happen next.

"PMS is the most provocative of all diseases. It'd be nice to have cancer, it'd be nice to have heart disease, because then you could point to it and you could go to a hospital and they could do something about it. And somebody says, 'How come you feel so lousy?' You can say, 'Oh, I've got cancer.' That's so much infinitely easier to explain than to say, 'Well, I just feel like heck. I don't feel good. I don't behave well today.' What do you say?

"Well, for the women here, now you know you have PMS and suddenly you know you're not crazy, that this is a *physical* problem. It's a chemical problem, and you're not insane.

"For the husbands, it's difficult to deal with. If some guy rams your new car and you get out and you discover that the guy had an epileptic seizure while he was driving down the street and couldn't help himself, that's fine, that helps you understand the guy who rammed your car. But it doesn't do anything for your car. So the domestic discord is easier to understand if you've got a wife with PMS, but it doesn't make the suffering any easier. What I'm suggesting to you is that there are some ways that you can help, husbands.

"One is that you know that it's physical. Keep telling yourself that over and over again. Two is know that your wife can't help herself. No matter how much positive thinking you give her, no matter how many self-control pep talks you give her, she can't help it. There's nothing she can do. And so if she can't do it, you have to. And that, my friends, is tough. It's tough! Because dealing with these women is no simple thing. Remember, don't blame them; don't pass along the guilt because the guilt is deep enough and thick enough.

"Take the kids, if you can, when Mom's that way. Take the kids out to the car and say, 'Let's go to the zoo.' Or take them into their room and read them a story. Let her sleep in the morning, get the kids off to school in the morning, take care of them if you can. Better still, give the wife the key to the car and say, 'You go to the zoo.' Because she needs time away. If you have a cabin, a condominium, a grandmother with a spare room, a basement, give her the key to it, let her get out of your life for a little while, and say, 'Go away for a couple of days.' She can't deal with people, and especially she can't deal with people she loves because the guilt is more than she can handle. You've got to try to protect them."

Chapter 10

"... work at least gives him a secure place in a portion of reality, in the human community."

Sigmund Freud, Civilization and Its Discontents

On the Job

Work defines us; we are what we do. Traditionally, women managed the household and raised the children. The homemaker, the housewife, the mother were the classic definitions of a woman. Today, nearly forty-eight million American women work outside the home in full-time jobs of every type and intensity. The definition of woman is now all-encompassing, whether blue-collar, pink-collar, or white-collar: clerk-typist or executive, lab technician or physician, assembly-line worker or factory owner, waitress or caterer, engineer, truck driver, television producer. Women can do everything. They prove it every day. Most of those forty-eight million American women are also married and the mothers of children. They're doing it all. But at great personal expense.

Economic survival has always been the primary reason that people work. That hasn't changed. Sheer necessity, not love of labor, created instant workforces for coal mines, oilfields, steel mills, textile plants, and auto factories. Despite the revolution in attitudes forced by the women's movement, in fact, the majority of American women work outside the home because they have to support themselves or children or because the family can't survive without two incomes.

But the beliefs that shape our approach to work have changed dramatically over the years. As William Faulkner once said: "You can't eat for eight hours a day nor drink for eight hours a day nor make love for eight hours a day — all you can do for eight hours is work. Which is the reason why man makes himself and everybody else so miserable and unhappy."

The work ethic on which this nation was founded no longer has much influence on how or why we work. The view that a man or woman becomes a better person by virtue of the act of working has been superseded by the more compelling thirst for ego satisfaction and personal recognition. It's a thirst that some women, especially those new to a career and eager to make their mark, seem unable to slake. As Studs Terkel wrote in the introduction to his book, *Working*, work is a search "for daily meaning as well as daily bread, for recognition as well as cash, for astonishment rather than torpor; for a sort of life rather than a Monday through Friday sort of dying." But he says, work is also "by its very nature, about violence — to the spirit as well as to the body... To survive the day is triumph enough for the walking wounded among the great many of us... The scars, psychic as well as physical, brought home to the supper table and the TV set, may have touched, malignantly, the soul of our society."

Women who work usually invest more of themselves, more of their identity, in a job or project than men do. They tend to care more, to take it all more personally than men. This is both an advantage and a disadvantage. It may bring women higher psychic rewards when they perform well and are recognized for their production. But their very personal stake in a job can magnify any disappointment or setback that might occur.

Women with severe premenstrual syndrome find their lives so disrupted by mood changes, depression, outbursts of temper, or physical discomfort that their work is affected. Stress exacerbates the syndrome, which is why women who are managing a household and raising children in addition to holding down a job, and high-achieving women in demanding professions tend to have the most extreme episodes of PMS. The pressure on today's women can reach inhuman levels. Expectations of women in our society, from hearth to boardroom, are three or four times higher than they are for men. To excel at everything, fulfill all responsibilities, personal and professional, and compete in a marketplace whose male-designed, but unwritten gameplans they've only recently begun to fathom — these are burdens that most men do not face. And if they did, men would probably refuse to assume them. Like sorority pledges and first-season rookies, women feel compelled to shoulder big loads without complaint while they "prove" themselves; they don't think they've earned the privilege, the luxury, of saying "enough."

This superwoman complex is a destructive phenomenon. No one can be all things to all people in all circumstances. By setting unattainable goals and marathon schedules, women set themselves up for failure: not because of inability but an overload of capacity. This is where stress comes in. Stress makes any health problem worse. It can cause infections to flare up and bring on headaches. During a stressful situation the body must mobilize so many of its systems to prepare for a crisis or attack or injury that any weak spot in the body breaks down. In women troubled by PMS, symptoms that might otherwise remain dormant or appear as mild warning signals suddenly rage out of control. When an episode of PMS affects a woman's work — if she loses her temper with a client or has a crying spell in front of her co-workers — the ramifications are far-reaching. Her behavior during a premenstrual phase can change the image of a woman in the eyes of her employer, manager, peers, or clients. Even more damaging is the impact of such incidents on the woman's self-esteem and sense of worth. I am what I do is not just a catch phrase. Most people, certainly most Americans, identify themselves with their work. To perform well bolsters self-image and self-confidence; it's a motivating force for even greater professional and personal accomplishment. To fail to live up to one's expectations on the job or to fall into disfavor with a boss or co-worker can be as devastating as rejection by a lover; it strikes at one's sense of self. When a woman's PMS symptoms emerge in the workplace, growing more frequent and more serious, she'll lose confidence in her abilities. She may become indecisive and unable to meet deadlines. Ultimately, untreated, she is likely to develop a major clinical depression.

About sixty percent of the more than two thousand patients we've evaluated work outside the home. Almost all of these women say that PMS has affected their work negatively; it would be surprising if it didn't. A major health problem will affect anyone's job performance, male or female. A man with severe arthritis couldn't juggle as many responsibilities as most women do who have serious PMS. But women afflicted with premenstrual syndrome adapt, sometimes with great ingenuity. The vast majority of our patients have managed successfully to work, maintain personal relationships, and raise their children, despite the presence in their lives each month of a debilitating illness. They have developed the most highly sophisticated coping mechanisms we have ever seen in any group of men or women. The media's image of women with PMS sometimes has been that of immature or incompetent women who fumble through life or can't control themselves. That's a highly inaccurate picture, bearing as much resemblance to reality as a sawhorse to a thoroughbred.

Women with PMS are experts at managing stress; they've done it with one hand tied behind their back for years.

Premenstrual syndrome raises different problems for different women. For some, it affects their memory and concentration, and makes it difficult for them to organize data or meet deadlines. For Roseanne Macri, a national sales director of a Los Angeles company, memory was the weak point. "Once a week every month, I would blank. I could not remember phone numbers. That would drive me up a wall because I'm capable of memorizing over two hundred companies and telling you exactly what was in their display at a show. I realize now that just before the final phase of the symptoms I'm not able to hear properly and I'm not able to grasp what people are saying. People I work with realize I'm that way at that time now, so they're more tolerant, they speak more slowly."

Val Peters, an office manager in Atlanta, recalls, "I couldn't concentrate or focus on things in the office. Getting a piece of paper out of the file would fluster me. I work with figures and budgets; it gets quite complicated. I remember when I first started, my boss would explain things to me and I'd realize that I had no idea what he was talking about. I couldn't concentrate. It was uncomfortable and frustrating. I'd also argue with my co-workers over trivial things. Normally I'm fairly mild-mannered, but before my period I'd get real irritable. Some days I would pass people in the hall and I wouldn't look them in the eye because I couldn't bring myself to say hello. It was like I'd become anti-people. Everyone irritated me. What's really shocking is that I could remember the exact moment that it would lift. That same afternoon I'd walk down the hall and greet the same people that I ignored that morning. I'd feel bad, like I should apologize for being unfriendly. There was such a strong contrast in the way I felt. I never asked whether anyone noticed the change in me because I was so ashamed of the way I felt. But when I asked one of the secretaries in the office to help me with my charting [she lives alone], she said, 'You've been very quiet during that week or so.' I hid the way I was feeling, I guess, but it was very strong internally.''

Dr. Glynis Morgan, forty-two, is the divorced mother of two college-age sons, who heads a major department of a large urban medical center. She had had mild symptoms since the birth of her first child, when she had postpartum depression for six months. Eight years ago she developed ''periodic paralysis,'' a profound muscle weakness that her physicians could not find explain. Her thighs actually became paralyzed about three times before her period; the paralysis lasted about twelve hours. After a tubal ligation in 1979, however, she began to experience irritability, breast pain, and depression, in addition to her other symptoms. Having PMS did affect her career, she says, but not as dramatically as it might have because her major health complaints did not begin until she had achieved a position of authority. ''I've done everything that I could have done, but it's been very difficult because of the physical symptoms. I didn't have the energy or the stamina that I should have had. I don't think that if I felt the whole time like I did those last three times that I could have done all that I did. I feel tremendous sympathy for young women who are starting out [in their careers] and have to deal with PMS, too.'' Progesterone makes her feel ''remarkably better. It's all the difference in the world.''

Our patients often say they were unable to produce a report on time because they couldn't synthesize the material or write a cohesive paragraph, or that they felt that their efficiency and productivity was sharply diminished during their symptom days. Nancy Winston, sales manager of a high-technology company in Silicon Valley, complained that she could only make sales calls three weeks a month; during the fourth week she went into the office, but limited her activity to administrative work and phone calls. Since she started treatment at the clinic, she's able to make outside sales calls all month long and has increased her sales commissions and productivity by more than twenty-five percent. Another woman, a key executive of a large Asian import business, had a similar problem; her employer was so concerned — and she was so valuable to his company — that he helped locate our center and bought her airline ticket to Boston to make certain she was treated.

Her symptoms have also been eliminated by progesterone therapy.

In some cases, colleagues and employers of the women who say their work quality varies cyclically disagree; they say these women are valued employees whose work is consistently of very high quality. We realize that some of the problems and fears our patients relate about their job performance are in fact just that. They feel less efficient, indecisive, confused, disoriented, unable to concentrate, but their boss or co-workers don't notice a drop in the quality of their performance. These women usually manage to control their symptoms until after they leave work. Still, that haunting sense of unease on the job is psychologically damaging; if untreated for too long, it inevitably results in actual problems at work.

A large number of our patients completed college and earned a bachelor's degree but were forced to withdraw from graduate school or decided not to enroll because PMS so affected their memory and concentration that they couldn't keep up with the more demanding work loads. A few women say they decided not to pursue medical careers because they knew they couldn't handle the demands of medical school and a hospital residency. Still others report that they have refused promotions because they didn't feel they could handle more responsibility and PMS, too. An attorney in Chicago says she changed law firms four times in nine years, at least twice because of PMS. The last move was to a firm that wanted to make her a partner. She finally convinced the managing partner that she was only interested in a commitment to the firm as a senior associate.

Some women say they grow suspicious or paranoid of others during their premenstrual phase. A producer of a major network television show says she spent most of her time in her office during her week of symptoms, with the excuse that she needed to catch up on paperwork. She wouldn't socialize with fellow employees, grew very distrustful of other people's motives, and agonized over imaginary errors. At one point, completely without reason or evidence, she believed her work was being criticized and that her boss was about to fire her. In talking to her co-workers, however, we were told she was and is a very valuable employee.

PMS women are the chameleons of the workplace; they are superb adapters. To cope with their symptoms and manage to get their jobs done, whenever possible, they schedule travel, difficult negotiations, critical contract discussions, and the start and completion of important projects for their good days. One literary agent confessed to handling book negotiations and sales only during her normal weeks and scheduling calls to publishers about overdue advance and royalty payments to her clients when she was "feeling bitchy." An attorney for a large Washington D.C. firm has a similar strategy. "I never make decisions or close deals on my premenstrual days. Those days I reserve for paperwork and thrashing out difficult points with difficult lawyers for the other side. Interestingly, I usually get my way."

PMS Leads to Absenteeism

Increased absenteeism is a byproduct of premenstrual syndrome. Many, but not all, of our patients say they occasionally or frequently stay home from work when they are unable to function or feel out of control. A typical history is that of Charity Evans, thirty-two, who teaches comparative literature at a Southern college. She says, "I miss one day of work about every other month. Every missed work day was because of cramps. I felt so bad that I couldn't go in. When I managed to make it in, I didn't do as good a job as I could have. Sometimes I felt as if I were going to lose control." She also experienced mild anxiety attacks; they were never so severe that she had to leave her classroom. "I just had to be strong and bear with the symptoms. I didn't want to give in to them."

Women have a forty-three percent higher absenteeism rate than men; PMS may be one factor but childcare and household responsibilities is known to be another. According to the Bureau of Labor Statistics, women were absent from their jobs because of illness or injury 4.3 percent of usual hours worked in 1981 compared with 3.0 percent for men. According to BLS, "The difference appears to be linked in part with family responsibilities of married women. The rate for single women was about the same as that for all men." A Labor Department study, "Absent Workers and Lost Hours," published in May 1978, noted, "Married women reported a higher proportion of time off for both illness and injury and miscellaneous personal reasons than did single women." One study reported that thirty-six percent of fifteen hundred women in one industrial plant sought sedation in the premenstrual week and may have lowered productivity as a result. A 1969 estimate put the cost to industry of absenteeism due to PMS at $5 billion; adjusting that estimate to 1982 dollars would raise the figure to nearly $10 billion.

Chronic absences exact a price; women may be reprimanded by their boss or fired. One woman's employer finally asked her for a letter from her physician about the causes of her frequent absences. Her physician gave her a lot of tests but told her she was normal and wouldn't support her claim of illness. She managed to negotiate a compromise with her employer by promising to miss no more days of work. Women in this situation, pressured to fulfill commitments they can't handle, begin to try to the hide their premenstrual problems. This adds to the stress, which worsens the symptoms.

Accident Rates Rise, Too

Studies show that more women have accidents in their premenstrual days than at other times. For some women, especially those in blue-collar or industrial jobs, this tendency can be downright dangerous. Patty Clemens, twenty-eight, a truck driver in Ohio, began experiencing a range of symptoms after undergoing a tubal ligation three years ago, including dizziness, cramps, confusion, anxiety, headaches, "funny" vision, spaciness, impairment of judgment and concentration. She's had several accidents and near-misses on the road during her premenstrual phase. "It would really get wild. Driving a large truck in city traffic is stressful to begin with. When I had my period, everything was magnified a hundred times. If someone cut me off three days before I got my period, I'd want to run him off the road." She said that she had accidents every Friday before her period for the three months before she came to our center for treatment. "I was so distracted, I couldn't think as quickly as I usually could. I'd lost my quickness of thought." She tore the side off a sports car on the first Friday. On the second, "a construction truck cut through my truck. It wasn't my fault, but I could have avoided it if I had been thinking more quickly." On the third Friday, a cab driver rounded a corner and rammed into her truck. "I felt so spaced out that I couldn't react."

Emotional outbursts are one of the most common reactions of women with premenstrual syndrome. Judy Firella, a microbiologist for a pharmaceutical company in New Jersey, had a classic case of depression and irritability that had gotten worse since the birth of her two children. "I felt as if I were on the top of a roller coaster, and I knew that I'd have to go all the way down to the bottom of the hill." She is troubled by the impact she feels PMS has had on her career: "I'd overreact. I'd get too emotional." She remembers one day when her boss brought a "filthy dirty desk, from a bar," into her pristine laboratory. She says she screamed at him for fifteen minutes, following him around the lab and into his office, complaining about the dirt and contamination the desk carried. Then she stalked out of his office, slamming the door behind her. He called after her, "Hey, you, come back." But she didn't. She says that she was always justifiably angry, but she didn't handle her anger "in a professional manner."

Cathie St. James, thirty-eight, single, no children, is a management consultant, whose work involves writing, organizing seminars and study projects. "I was so fatigued during those two weeks that I didn't have the mental ability to do my work, and I noticed that my production was dropping. I could do the reports that I had to do, but I had no mental energy for creative writing. I've never missed a seminar, or even an appointment, no matter how bad I felt. Other people may have been debilitated by my condition, but my upbringing and my conditioning wouldn't allow me to skip work." She says that her irritability sometimes spilled over into anger, but never at the office. "Sometimes when I got home from work, I'd lose control. I broke dishes, I broke a radio, but I always broke things instead of people." She feels that if she hadn't been so self-disciplined, she might have become violent. She has a very rigid physical routine for herself: She runs six to eight miles every day and lifts weights and does body building exercises every day as well. During those two weeks, however, she found it difficult to run even two miles, although she did force herself to do the two miles.

Claudia Sorano, a bank vice president in Chicago, handles major accounts and gets high ratings from her superiors. Except that they have noted that periodically she overreacts to stressful situations with anger and irritability. This has happened half a dozen times in the bank, but on at least two occasions that were memorable. Once she and several colleagues were out of town negotiating a major loan. The attorney for the client made a critical comment that she would normally have overlooked or diplomatically glossed over. Instead, she launched into a tirade against the man. Luckily one of her colleagues smoothed it over and the deal was completed. But later her colleague took her aside and reprimanded her, saying "You almost blew it for us." She felt terrible because she knew that she was premenstrual, that she should have kept her mouth shut, but she couldn't control herself.

Later she got promoted to another division and during one of the weekly meetings of vice presidents a similar thing happened. Another vice president made a seemingly innocuous comment and she took offense, letting loose verbally. Her boss noted it and later cautioned her that she couldn't behave that way. She knew her harangue was inappropriate. Soon after this she came to us for evaluation; she had known about PMS but had been denying it until the second incident.

Jill Morton, an architect for a large California design firm, first became aware of her PMS at work: "People who are close to you and personally involved with you tend to accept your problems more than people you work with." Several times, she says, her condition interfered with her nascent career. "In two specific incidents, my behavior became uncontrollable. Once with a customer, once with a person I worked for. I behaved very poorly. I lost my temper. I said a lot of things — that perhaps were true — that I would never have said under normal circumstances. I just said, 'Look, this is what is going to happen, buzz out of this situation, here I am and I'm taking over.' Mostly to superiors. This was interesting because I was in a program where I was evaluated very closely, in terms of advancement. One of my last evaluations was that I had very many strong points but that my inability was that I became so intense that I lost control of my temper. I lost control of the situation because I tend to overreact. Mostly I lashed out verbally. I've only thrown things at my husband, nobody else. Never at work. You don't throw things at guys who pay you."

Morton feels that her natural candor and aggressiveness is dramatically magnified when she is premenstrual. "I think that people recognize that I can do certain things, but they also feel that I am extremely volatile and that in certain circumstances they prefer to have someone else handle it if it's a very political type of situation, because I may lose my temper. I may tell the truth where they... I may be too painfully candid. What people think of me is that I'm very aggressive. In certain situations it's too much, in others, it's very good. I think it's hurt me in certain instances, but banking is a career that today accepts a certain amount of aggressiveness. Yet women who are aggressive are sometimes looked on as somewhat of a shocking element and they [men] don't know how to react.''

Problems in the Classroom

School teachers with premenstrual syndrome have classroom outbursts, and are less flexible and tolerant of the students' behavior. One patient even considered giving up teaching because she couldn't handle the stress, and felt she was being unfair to her classes. But she got treatment, eliminated her symptoms, and continued with her teaching career. Patty Montand, a thirty-nine-year-old high school teacher, says: ''When you teach, you need total control. The week before my period, I would feel as if I were going to explode. I was so irritable that I would take it out on the students.'' Twice parents came in for conferences after she verbally abused a student. ''All I could say was that I was sorry. I didn't know what was going on myself.'' Thinking back, she's amazed it didn't happen more often. ''I was never physically violent with the kids, but I was hostile and verbally abusive. It was always an overreaction on my part if they talked in class, or if they came in late.''

Lucy Romano, thirty-two, was a school principal until her problems with PMS made her decide to go back to graduate school and finish her doctorate. ''I'm very good with kids, but before I'd get my period I'd lose control and yell at them.'' When a student was sent to her office for disciplinary action during the wrong time of month, she would get irrationally angry. ''I would take it too seriously. If I had to do one more thing than I had planned to do that day, it would set me off.'' She said, ''I'm bright, mature, responsible and all that. When I would react like this, I thought that I was losing my mind.'' One day she went to work feeling terrible. She remembers telling herself, ''Just stay calm. Walk into your office and control yourself.'' When she got in, she slammed her office door and broke down in tears. She went to see the superintendent of the school district, told him she had menstrually-related problems, and said, ''I can't do it. Just send me home for a week.'' She took the week off, but when she returned, the superintendent ''didn't trust me anymore. He didn't think that I could handle the job, and he kept me from proving myself by preventing me from handling all the responsibilities that I should have." She describes her job as stressful. "They replaced me with two and a half people."

For some reason, we've treated a relatively large number of professional singers over the past three years, especially opera singers. Sandra Condon, forty-one, is a part-time opera singer and administrative assistant. The PMS affected her singing. "It takes a lot of energy to sing," she says. "I'd be too tired, and too unmotivated. And I didn't sing well two weeks before my period, and the week of my period. I really could sing well only seven days of the month." When she felt well, she would sing some scales before dinner, and sing songs and exercises after dinner. She sings fifteen minutes out of every hour: Bellini and Handel arias, Italian art songs. She was offered the leading role in Gilbert and Sullivan's *Princess Ida,* but she took a secondary role instead because of her PMS. The performance was scheduled for the day her period would start. "I knew that I wouldn't be able to sing high Bs that night." When women menstruate, she said, their voices drop down a part of an octave. Her performance went well, but "I couldn't have sung the lead role." She remembers singing in a lieder class during the spring of 1980. "It was a couple of days before my period. I just had to get up and sing a couple of German songs; it was really no big deal. But I remember getting up and wishing that I wasn't there. I was very depressed. I got through the songs, but without the flair I normally would have."

Opting for Flexible Schedules

About half of our patients who work have changed their job circumstances or quit work or school to cope with PMS. Consulting and freelance work is one of the most common choices of working women with PMS because of the flexibility of schedules it offers. Many women decide to give up simply to avoid confrontations.

Marguerite Sorenson, thirty-nine, is an artist who lives in Maine with her husband and two teenage sons. She worked as a commercial artist for an advertising agency until five years ago when her health problems grew difficult. Sorenson is glad that she had the flexibility as an artist to work at home, but her illness jeopardized her career, making it tough for her to meet her commitments. But her painting helped her to cope with her pain and depression. Her specialty is representational work in watercolor — landscapes, flowers and nature scenes. Her work reflects her feelings and emotions. "When I was feeling terrible, I would use a lot of dark colors."

Amy Dorfman, thirty-eight, the mother of two sons, has quit three jobs in seven years because of PMS, as a market researcher, magazine advertising salesperson, and caterer. The first two jobs she left with "impulsive, emotional resignations" caused by incidents that occurred during her premenstrual phase. On the first job, she said she had been owed money for two or three months. When the office manager walked around distributing checks to her coworkers, but she was not paid, she lost her temper and screamed at the office manager. "I made an absolute fool of myself in front of four people who worked for me." Her boss took her aside and talked to her, telling her that she was disappointed in her reaction. Dorfman cried during the talk, and quit in anger. Her boss asked her to stay with the firm, and offered to double her salary but she refused. "I was so ashamed of myself, and I was afraid that I'd do the same thing again." While she was employed by the catering company, she didn't show up for work for one week. "I felt as if I couldn't cope. My husband was away, and I took the children and went to stay with a friend. I didn't call my boss or tell him that I was leaving. When I returned to the office the following week, he was very understanding, but again, I was so ashamed that I resigned." At her sales job, "I was a terrifically qualified, hard worker at times. And at other times, I just fell apart. There were days where I'd go in and pull lists of calls to make and they'd swim in front of me. I'd go in two hours early, because I knew that I had client appointments all day and I felt so disorganized. But I was so disoriented that the extra two hours really didn't help." Dorfman called in with the flu a lot, but "I'd force myself to go to work as much as I could because to stay home alone would be devastating. I'd be so depressed that I'd go to pieces. I'd get dressed, put on my makeup and try to hang in there, no matter how difficult it was." She never missed a client appointment when she was working, but in the summer of 1981 she took three weeks off. "I talked to my boss. Actually, I sat there and cried. She suggested that I take some time off and relax." She forced herself to do things. "I forced myself to go to work, and I forced myself to go to parties. I was more capable of forcing myself to get things done on the outside. The worst times were when I was home and I didn't have much to do.'' Dorfman eventually told the sales staff she worked with — all women — about PMS after an article about it ran in a leading newsmagazine and she felt that she could be treated. ''They were understanding,'' and allowed her to rearrange the days that she would work in the office. ''They told me that they could tell when it was a week or two before my period just by looking at me. I'd look extremely strained and white, as if I were under a lot of stress.''

Dealing With Anxiety Attacks

Some women report having panic attacks or incidents with phobias when PMS combines with the stress of a high-pressure job. One sales person for a computer company had panic attacks related to driving a car. As a sales person who made calls on clients, this interfered with her work. ''During those two weeks, I would experience an absolute terror of driving. I did drive, but I was scared to death that I'd have an accident. I'd stay off the parkways, and I couldn't drive in the city because I couldn't maintain anything near the average speed.''

Lola Scott, a real estate broker, relates an incident in the summer of 1981, ''that was my nightmare period, just before I got treatment. I was supposed to run an open house. That's where the listing sales person serves lunch for the other brokers in the area and shows them the house that is up for sale. There was a terrible thunderstorm the night before that woke me up at three in the morning. It poured with rain all day. I packed the food in the car and took the kids to drop them off at a friend's house. I was dressed in a pretty dress in the car with the food and the children, and the roads were flooded. There were stalled cars everywhere. I reacted totally irrationally. I saw myself stuck in a puddle forever. I got hysterical and said things like 'I'm never going to get there.' I knew that the open house wasn't that important, that if I were having trouble getting there, so was everyone else. The kids were great. 'No, Mom, everything's going to be okay,' my son said. 'Why don't you take this road instead?' And all I could do was see myself stuck in that puddle, in my pretty dress, with the kids and the food in the trunk of the car, forever.''

A magazine editor in New York had her first panic attack when stuck in a subway tunnel. She had been writing and making notes on manuscripts when the train suddenly got stuck in the tunnel; she was one day away from her period. Eventually the passengers had to leave the subway and walk out through the tunnel. Since then she hasn't been able to force herself to ride the subway, and has spent a small fortune on cabs. She subsequently had several other panic attacks and was treated with psychotherapy, but it didn't work. We first saw her as a patient for treatment of the panic attack. In checking her medical history, though, we saw that she had several other cyclical complaints, all of which had been getting worse in recent years. Since she's been treated with progesterone she has not experienced any cyclical symptoms in the premenstrual time. But she's still in therapy for her fear of subways and tunnels.

Keeping PMS Under Wraps

Few women in positions of authority have discussed their cyclical problem with anyone connected to their job, although a few of our patients in lower-level jobs say they have discussed PMS with co-workers. Very rarely a woman will have told a superior about her condition. Group leaders for the National PMS Society say women who call for referrals to support groups in their area frequently say they are afraid to mention PMS at work for fear of being fired or having their responsibilities diminished; they're also afraid to file claims for reimbursement of medical expenses with their employer's insurance company for fear that PMS will somehow reflect upon them or affect their job status.

Jill Morton, the architect, takes the majority view: "I think that probably the hardest thing is to admit, at least in a professional capacity, that you are afflicted with this thing. I would never say at work that I had PMS. I would feel my working associates, mostly men, would say, 'Aha. Raging hormones. We always knew.' It's the kind of thing that's like a closet sickness. I have to go to the doctor, and if I said it was for my toe, they would say, 'Oh, yeah. That's really bad.' But if you say I have this problem because I have a hormone imbalance and when I get my period it makes me really miserable. People are uncomfortable with that kind of a biological discussion while they're not if you broke your toe or your finger. I've not at all indicated my PMS in a professional capacity. Because I feel that people who are in the position of power right now are not in a position to understand something like that. It's something that's relatively new. The people for whom I work are from a generation that never spoke of those things.''

Education about premenstrual syndrome, its physiological basis, and the availability of treatment should one day erase the stigma that many women feel attaches to their condition. The recent emergence of interest in premenstrual syndrome is a natural outgrowth of the dramatic rise in the number of women in the workforce. As women have moved out into careers, developing complex and demanding professional, political, and social roles, they have reached a stage where they can't and won't tolerate the illness and its interference in their lives any longer. Society's emphasis on health education and prevention, nutrition, exercise, and management of stress has made women more sensitive, aware, and demanding about their physical well-being. They're now vocal advocates for sensible, intelligent health care and refuse to be dictated to by physicians or anyone else who can't resolve their medical complaints.

Chapter 11

Violence is here,
In the world of the sane,
And violence is a symptom.

Jacob Bronowski, **The Face of Violence**

Striking Out

Lizzie Borden hated her stepmother with a steely white-hot intensity that had mounted without pause for five years. It was undoubtedly the profoundest emotion that Abby Durfee Borden had ever stirred in another. At sixty-five, Abby was dismal and uninteresting, a two-hundred-pound semi-recluse with few interests and less imagination. What she did have was a husband, Andrew J. Borden, Lizzie's seventy-year-old father and president of the local bank. Jealousy and greed fueled Lizzie's hatred and had ever since Andrew had purchased for Abby a half-interest in her sister's house for $1,500. The gift was Abby's only real asset; it was the only major sum of money transferred from husband to wife. And it detracted not one whit from Lizzie or her sister Emma. Both of them were well provided for by their father, both had their own checking and savings accounts, and income from real estate in their own names. Lizzie, Andrew's favorite despite her erratic nature, had at the time of her trial more than $3,000 in her own right, an enormous sum then for a thirty-two-year-old single woman. But Lizzie wanted more; most of all she wanted her father out of Abby's grasp. She certainly didn't want Abby to gain further from her father's wealth.

Sometime in the spring or summer of 1892 Lizzie Borden learned of a plan of her father's that outraged her. He intended to secretly transfer the ownership of his Swansea farm to Abby prior to letting John Morse, the brother of his deceased first wife, take over Swansea and its expenses as a kind of caretaker/boarder. The secrecy was intended to prevent Lizzie and Emma from finding out that Abby now owned two properties. Lizzie apparently never confronted her father with her discovery. Instead, by July, she was actively planning to kill Abby, to poison her with an untraceable substance. Lizzie made the rounds of Fall River's drugstores trying to buy prussic acid, to no avail. Pharmacists told her that prussic acid, a highly volatile and dangerous element, was not sold without a prescription. Later, a policeman noticed that the spine of the family's book of household hints was broken; its pages opened naturally to the section on prussic acid. Lizzie's lack of subtlety at the drug counters and with the household hints apparently alerted Abby to her plans; if Lizzie had known enough about poison to ask for arsenic she would have readily obtained it and would never have become an American legend.

After the tantrums and outcry Lizzie had kindled over the $1,500 house interest, Abby feared Lizzie intensely, terribly, and with good reason. Two days before the murders, after the Bordens en masse and their Irish maid Bridget Sullivan suffered bouts of nausea and vomiting, Abby ran to the home of a physician-neighbor telling him she had been threatened by poison and then poisoned in fact. She conveniently ignored the likely tie of the illness to a family meal of leftover fish following three days of mutton, probably tainted by the August weather. The physician, however, inquired into the Borden menus and assured her that the cause of the complaints was summer food poisoning. That night, Lizzie visited her friend Alice Russell, and described "this feeling as if something was hanging over me that I cannot shake off." The aura of temporal epilepsy was wafting over her; one of Lizzie's "peculiar spells" was coming on.

An Oppressive Dawn

By dawn of the following day, Thursday, August 4, 1892, an oppressive shroud of heat and humidity hung over Fall River; it was to be the hottest day in memory for several decades in a town distinguished by its wilting summers. It was also the first day of Lizzie Borden's menstrual flow. Despite the recent outbreak of unsettled stomachs, the household — Andrew and Abby Borden, Uncle John Morse, and Bridget — took a dining room breakfast of mutton, mutton broth, bananas, cookies, and johnnycakes. Lizzie, showing better sense, or perhaps preoccupied with her work at hand, chose coffee and cookies in the kitchen. After breakfast, Uncle John left on an errand; Bridget went outside to wash windows, following Abby's instructions; Andrew djourned to the bank, where he planned to meet Abby and deed over he Swansea property to her. Abby went upstairs to the guest room, elling Lizzie she was going to put fresh slipcovers on the pillows on the ed that also served as a couch. The opportunity must have seemed eaven-sent. No one was in the house except Abby and Lizzie. But what appened next defied logic.

Lizzie slipped down to the cellar and grabbed a hatchet, bringing it p to the kitchen. The doorbell rang. A messenger delivered a note for Abby, probably a last minute exhortation and reassurance from Andrew hat she should meet him at the bank, that Lizzie and Emma would not liscover the transaction. Giddy with the realization that her plan was bout to be set irrevocably in motion, Lizzie called up to Abby that a nessage had arrived for her and that she would carry it up with the wash. Arranging a pile of clean clothes to hide the ax, Lizzie clutched the inens, and ascended the staircase to the guestroom. As Abby Borden traightened up from smoothing the bedspread, Lizzie moved up behind ter, and in one gesture, pulled the hatchet free as she flung the clothes away. With a single well-placed stroke, she laid Abby out unconscious, robably dead. Taking a moment to fasten the window's wooden hutters, she proceeded to bludgeon her stepmother nineteen more times — in what one physician termed "weak and ill-aimed blows for a nan."

Without question, Lizzie had planned to kill Abby. But the murder tself and the subsequent murder of her father, whom she loved dearly, vere probably committed in an episode of premenstrual syndrome. Her rimary symptom was recurring epileptic seizures of the temporal lobe, robably marked by automatism — a period of automatic action in which the victim may remember only dimly or may forget completely ter actions during the seizure, as Victoria Lincoln describes it in *A Private Disgrace — Lizzie Borden by Daylight*. Abby Durfee Borden vas a murder target, but she was probably a victim of Lizzie's PMS and pilepsy. The conscious Lizzie had chosen a woman's means of killing — poison. She didn't want to create a mess. She didn't want to get :aught. In the sleep-walker's motion that is automatism, Lizzie reached 'or a distinctly masculine weapon — an ax — that was at once too olatant, too obvious, too bloody a method for her nature. There's no question of the cause of death when a hatchet's involved; gashes and gaping wounds can't be blamed on rancid mutton. Victoria Lincoln believes that Lizzie's seizure ended "when that orgasm of hate was spent." After dealing death to Abby, she emerged from the haze of the epileptic automatism, saw the clothes still clean on the floor behind her, was stunned to find blood on her hands. Then she did what any pragmatic murderer would do: she cleaned herself up, stashed the ax in a tall slop pail nearby, and slipped downstairs as if everything were normal.

The Fatal Mistake

She had ample time to create a situation that could make it appear that an unknown intruder, maybe a burglar, had entered the house and killed Abby. But a second surprise awaited her, one that forced her to change strategies rapidly. Her father returned home, an hour and a half before his normal lunch time. He was looking for Abby, although he couldn't tell Lizzie why. That was his fatal mistake. Even though the automatism had passed, by depriving Lizzie of the time and circumstances she needed to set up the discovery of Abby's body, Andrew Borden would die at the hands of his favorite daughter. Lizzie told Andrew that Abby had left to visit a friend; while that excuse didn't make much sense given Abby's tendency to stay within the boundaries of the house and yard, Andrew apparently accepted it at face value and decided to relax before lunch in the sitting room. He, too, was killed with the ax, but this time Lizzie, now more sure of herself, spent only ten blows on him as he napped on the parlor sofa.

Despite the predominance of the evidence and Lizzie's transparent and contradictory lies about the events of August 4, a jury of twelve gentlemen of Fall River acquitted her of both crimes. The bizarre murders remained a *cause celebre* long after the acquittal. Her exploits were exaggerated, as Americans are wont to do, in folk song and legend, telling of "forty whacks" for Abby and forty-one for her father.

Nearly a century later, Lawrence Sanders created another troubled and deadly woman, Zoe Kohler, in *The Third Deadly Sin*. Kohler, we learn, suffers from dysmenorrhea (extremely painful menstrual cramps), Addison's disease, premenstrual syndrome, and a number of psychoses that lead her to "act out" on the day before or the first day of menstruation. Not content to lose her temper or throw an ashtray again, a wall, Kohler marks her monthly cycle by killing; she kills men. In scenes far more grisly than those of the Borden household, the novel details the murders, one by one, of six men lured to bloody deaths in their hotel rooms.

Women and Violence

Neither Lizzie Borden nor the fictional Zoe Kohler murdered because of premenstrual syndrome; but both killed during episodes of PMS. In widely publicized instances, three women in England diagnosed as having PMS, convicted of killings during premenstrual episodes, received lenient sentences because of their illness. Despite the media play given to those three cases, examples of women out of control during experiences of premenstrual syndrome are extremely rare. That's hardly surprising since, to begin with, women account for a minority of the arrests and convictions for violent crimes and represent only one out of thirty prison sentences in this country. Women have accounted for only about fifteen percent of all murders since records have been kept; premenstrual syndrome could account for just a fraction of the total. Yet some violent acts committed by women may be the result of a specially heightened mood. During a research project on aggressive behavior in women conducted at a Massachusetts prison some years ago, we interviewed six women who were sentenced for murder — three victims were husbands, two were children, one was a lover. Two things that were striking about all six cases were that the killings occurred on the day before or first day of menstruation, and that all six women could have been described as quiet, mild-mannered housewives. As Enid Bagnold observed, "A murderess is only an ordinary woman in temper." That could be the temper of premenstrual syndrome.

Outbursts of anger, the throwing of objects, and on occasion even thoughts of murder are fairly common in women with PMS. A majority of women with PMS at some time or another, when under great stress or pain, say they have become angry, yelled, screamed, had a car accident, thrown something, or felt as if they wanted to throw something or act out against someone. Only ten to fifteen percent of the patients we have seen, however, have ever assaulted another person, their spouse or lover, or their children.

Links between menstruation and antisocial behavior were first made by criminologists in the 19th Century. The father of modern criminology, Italian scientist Cesare Lombroso and his son-in-law William Ferrero noted in their 1893 work *The Female Offender,* that of eighty women arrested for "resistance to public officials," seventy-one were menstruating. In 1890 S. Ikard cited a study of fifty-six Parisian shoplifters, of whom thirty-five were menstruating at the time of the offense. More than half a century later, another researcher quoted a French police prefect to the effect that eighty-four percent of female crimes of violence in Paris were perpetrated during the premenstrual and early menstrual phases of the cycle. Investigators who examined the behavior of women in prisons and special hospitals found they were more liable to aggressive behavior during the premenstrual and menstrual phases of their cycle. In 1953 Joseph Morton reported that the treatment of premenstrual tension in female prisoners resulted in improved behavior. In 1961 Dr. Katharina Dalton reported that forty-nine percent of one hundred fifty-six women convicted of theft, soliciting, and drunkenness committed the crimes just before or during menstruation. Of the forty-three women — twenty-seven percent — who complained of premenstrual symptoms, sixty-three percent committed their offenses at the time of their symptoms. The irascibility and tension that accompanies premenstrual symptoms makes some incidence of assaults and violence unavoidable, especially within families. As Jacob Bronowski wrote, "Violence is the sphinx by the fireside, and she has a human face."

Interviews with our patients yield hundreds of stories of incidents and outbursts, minor and major, related to PMS. "It was like being possessed," one woman remembers. "I'd fly at my husband, rip his jacket, smash his glasses. It was horrible and I was so ashamed."

With the cooperation of her husband and children, Carla Jones built up shelf upon shelf of glass jars and bottles in the family garage. When she felt a sense of rage rising and needed an outlet for it, she headed for the garage and smashed the glass against the floor, the wall, the driveway. Sometimes, she says, she'd stomp out to the garage in the wee hours of the morning, in robe and nightgown, and destroy a dozen or so jars. "It's the release of the urge to hit something that's important," Jones says. "It saves me the fear that I'll strike someone I love."

The Jones family concedes that the clean up is a little hazardous, and the glass is a danger to the tires on their two cars, but it's safer than any alternative.

Meg Newberry remembers being so upset one morning and feeling the aura of a migraine headache beginning that when her preschool daughter started to cry and wouldn't stop, she stalked into the child's bedroom to tell her to stop. "I was so furious and in such pain that I pushed the door incredibly hard and it bounced smack into the wall. I was so mad, I did it again and again. By the time I stopped I had punched a large hole in the plaster." She was chagrined later to discover that her daughter had a fever and the flu.

Incidents involving women with PMS and the men in their lives are fairly common, although few of them involve serious assaults or injuries. One patient, Tony Salazar, recalls her attempts to aggravate her husband, "I'd gun the car; I'd be so angry that he was afraid to let me drive. I'd bug him because I needed to do something with my anger." She threw pots, pans, dishes, glasses, "anything in reach." One day when she served dinner her husband looked at his plate and asked, "What is this garbage?" It was creamed corn, as he found out when she picked up his plate and threw it in his face.

While some women concede that they got physical with their mates or others they controlled their impulse for physical outbursts around their children. Nicole Maynard said her symptoms were so severe that she came close to hitting her three children, but never did. "I wouldn't touch them. I had enough control to stop myself. Although with my husband, he's a big guy, sometimes when I was really feeling bad, I'd start pounding on him."

Andrea Brixton, a thirty-six-year-old market researcher, is a soft-spoken divorced mother of three. She also found herself turning on other people. "I was violent toward others. My husband and I had marital problems for years, a lot of it because of my erratic behavior each month. Once I just decided I was going to kill myself with a kitchen knife, but I ended up stabbing him instead. He was in the hospital for a week with that. I had also slashed my wrists a few times before that."

Diana Robertson, thirty-nine, is a single schoolteacher. "I threw things," she says, "but only objects and never at a person, only around the room... Well, once I became terribly angry, explosive, and violent and I attacked my roommate with my fists. I didn't hurt her. But that kind of episode always happened in the two weeks prior to my period."

Leslie Talbot, twenty-eight, is a corporate benefits administrator; now divorced, she lives with a man and his three children. "I'm divorced because of PMS. I've been going through this for years. I don't want to get married again because of it. The first years my [current] friend and I were together, we could only live together half the month. Two weeks on and two weeks off. I've tried to kill him. I've tried to kill myself. More than once. It landed me in a sanitarium. Every time it was recorded that at the same time I had my period. The first two weeks of the month I'm an intelligent, reasonable person, and the second two I am a person completely out of control. Three weeks prior to my period — two weeks minimum — I become very over-anxious, depressed, and high-strung. It's as if all my emotions are pushed to the extreme. It's a constant mental battle to try to keep in control, and with all your effort going into that, it makes you understand what people say. It affects you physically. I broke glasses and bumped into things. I'm a freelance artist on weekends and in the evenings and I found I couldn't cut or draw a straight line during my symptoms. I didn't realize the clumsiness was a part of the syndrome. It's a complete physical change." She also has a hearing problem in the left ear that's worse in the premenstruum.

"There's another part of it. Because of the way you behave during PMS, people are mad at you, for having called them every name in the book. Since I've been treated, that part of it is gone. Things I used to neglect two weeks a month, I can now take care of steadily. I can maintain myself, so things around me are maintained. In my reactions, I have an opportunity to be normal. If I'm upset, I know it's for a reason, not because I'm suffering from PMS. And if I'm happy, it's not because I'm trying to be, it's real."

Debunking the Spouse Abuse Myth

Statistics on family assaults, between spouses or parent against child, are spotty at best. The attention paid in the late 1970s to the issue of battered husbands raised the possibility that spouse abuse by women may have been more frequent than attacks instigated by men, but men inflict the most serious physical damage.

Georganne Michaels focused her rage and depression on her husband, Peter, and sometimes their struggles escalated into violent brawls. Since Peter at 220 pounds is substantially larger and stronger than his wife, these encounters promised the most damage to Georganne. Peter Michaels recalls that "when the arguments started, they were over small, insignificant things... We'd have a small argument and she'd throw the wine in her glass at me. The argument would grow, and the glass would follow the wine." Once he locked her out of their bedroom. She took a hammer and tried "to bash down the bedroom door." In general, he says, "She'd be screaming and hysterical; I'd be trying to suppress this violent flailing animal.

"We'd have five-star, ocean-going rows and fights. I would be accused of things unjustly. I would try to fight back by sneering or walking around the house smiling — anything to reach the maximum boiling point in her. I'm a very big man, and I've played violent sports; I was afraid that I'd hit her. I cracked her ribs twice by holding her, when I was trying to restrain her and stop her struggling. Sometimes the difficulty of not picking up my fist and putting it into her face was an act of inhuman restraint."

Yet twice he lost such control. Once he came down to the kitchen and "she was bashing new Teflon frying pans against the counter. I thought they were coming at me next. When I held her, she struggled and when we moved next to the counter, I cracked her rib." When the second injury occurred, "I was lying in bed, and she jumped on top of me. I pulled her down, and my elbow went into her rib." Both times, he says, were accidents caused by "my considerable strength."

Certainly women with premenstrual syndrome may lash out at their husbands when angry and frustrated, but they are rarely the ones to inflict bodily harm. As Ann Jones points out in *Women Who Kill,* the contention of the main research paper on the subject, *The Battered Husband Syndrome* by Suzanne Steinmetz, that "husband-beating constitutes a sizeable proportion of marital violence" was not supported by the data; the Steinmetz study was subsequently roundly criticized by other scholars. The Steinmetz data actually showed roughly equal numbers of occasions when wives and husbands hit, pushed, and threw things. But, as Ann Jones notes, Steinmetz "overlooked the context of the events and left out altogether the types of physical attacks battered women most often experience... kicking, choking, cutting, bashing the head into a solid stationary object.'' In her work, Steinmetz cited criminologist Marvin Wolfgang's classic finding that wives killed their husbands almost as often as husbands killed their wives. She omitted Wolfgang's clarification that women were seven times more likely than the men to be acting in self-defense.

Rare Incidence of Child Abuse

Child abuse is another problem that remains largely hidden from public view. The true incidence of child abuse may never be known, but one assessment, extrapolated from the reporting rates of New York and Denver, is an average of two hundred fifty to three hundred cases a year per million residents. Others estimate that 0.2 percent of childhood injuries are caused by child abuse. In one study of hospitalizations of children, Dr. Dalton demonstrated a high rate of admissions of children for illness and accidents during the premenstrual phase of their mother's menstrual cycle. She has suggested that some cases of child abuse may be related to premenstrual tension but there have been no systematic studies. Among our patients, the incidence of child abuse is rare. But many of the women are extremely fearful that they might assault their children. Most incidents involving children that we hear of tend to be verbal. The mothers are hypercritical; a thirty-second scolding becomes a thirty-minute harangue. Usually when a woman feels a loss of control or an urge to strike a child, she'll walk away, out of the house, into the bedroom. It's the triumph of reason over emotion, requiring great restraint, that the women may not show with their husbands or lovers.

The kind of unexpected, apparently unprompted outbursts that Christina Crawford related about her mother, Joan Crawford, in *Mommie Dearest* go far beyond what most children with PMS mothers endure. But those graphic night raids, bursts of house cleaning and garden chores undertaken in the middle of the night, and unprovoked bouts of temper and imposition of punishments paint a picture of a woman with premenstrual syndrome. The most memorable scene from *Mommie Dearest* is, of course, the night raid involving the wire clothes hangers. ''Inside the closet my mother was in a rage. She was swearing a blue streak and muttering to herself... She grabbed me by the hair and dragged me into the closet. There before me I saw total devastation...

Shaking me by the hair she screamed in my ear, 'No wire hangers! No wire hangers!' With one hand she pulled me by the hair and with the other she pounded my ears until they rang and I could hardly hear her screaming.'' The loss of control and towering rage that Joan Crawford frequently exhibited are sensations shared by many women with PMS. Terry Wright, the mother of six children, is one of the rare women who admits that ''my first two kids were literally battered because I would just lose control.''

Lisa Santori, forty-three, describes the guilt she feels about the premenstrual violence that touched her three children, now grown and living on their own. ''I don't usually put my hands on my children. I'm not a person who normally hits children. I have and I will, but I do not believe in it. I was acting against my own beliefs but I couldn't control myself. Even now, they're twenty-five and twenty-six years old, and I realize that the things that I've done to them were probably at that time of the month. I just couldn't control myself, but I never related it to my period. I just thought they irritated me. As I learned about it, I realized that this is PMS and this is outside me. I mean I could tell the difference. I know the difference. After I'd do something I'd feel bad, and try to contain myself but that made me feel even worse. That sounds silly now. If I tried to contain myself it would be like trying to hold the flood back, the pressure would be a lot heavier. It was the same every month. The last three days before my flow, it was a nightmare for me.''

Doreen Trumbull's temper was more controlled but she remembers ''one spanking episode that was out of control'' and an incident in which ''I cuffed a stepchild around the face, which I shouldn't have done.'' In a large and boistrous household of two children belonging to both her husband and herself and five stepchildren from their previous marriages, strain and tension were a normal part of every weekend, she says. During one of those get-together Saturdays, Trumbull recalls, ''My husband and I ended up cuffing each other around'' over something minor, what a child had for dinner.

A frequent problem for these women are the feelings, the desire, to throttle or abuse a child. One women caller to a Phil Donahue television show about premenstrual syndrome said she often became enraged and out of control. Once she said she was about to throw her four-year-old through the living room picture window but she didn't because the

phone rang — it was her husband — and she went to answer it. There'
something to be said after all for the modern tyranny of the Bell System.

Two strategies developed by Veronica Minter, the mother of tw
preschoolers, redirected her anger. "I never got violent with the kids.
always kept myself back from them. But a few times, things would fly
across the room. If I felt like I could really kill the kids, I would beat
pillow against the wall. I would never really hurt them. But there were
times when I would grab the kids, throw them in the car, and go over to
somebody's house, because if I didn't get out of our house, I would be
them. I didn't want to do that. I really tried to protect them from me."

Chapter 12

*Dying
Is an art, like everything else.
I do it exceedingly well.*

Sylvia Plath, **Lady Lazarus**

Suicide Attempts

Suicide, like bizarre murders and the sex lives of celebrities, holds a morbid fascination for even the most civilized among us. Incidents of suicide, however horrifying, tantalize the closet voyeur and taunt us with the possibility that we, too, could take our own life. Killing oneself because of unbearable pressures, in the most depressed of states, is the picture most readily evoked by the word "suicide," but it is sometimes the outcome of a final nose-thumbing challenge. Tempting fate, like moths that fly too near a flame, is as deliberate a contest for some as a chess match. At stake is not an intricately carved knight, nor a queen, nor a king, but oneself. For these individuals "life loses interest," Freud wrote, "when the highest stake in the game of living, life itself, may not be risked." Whatever the trigger mechanism, the fatal attraction of suicide has long been evident. Centuries ago suicide was recognized as part of human frailty by church and state, which took drastic steps to caution the populace from even considering the taking of their own lives. Suicide was decreed a crime, a felony that in England and some other jurisdictions carried the ironic penalty of death. Dare suicide, the state thundered, and you'll regret it but not live. Englishmen who tried and failed during the 18th and 19th Centuries were revived just long enough to see the state undertake the deed in a much more efficient manner. The Roman Catholic Church deems suicide or the attempt a mortal sin, again bearing the same stigma and penalty as murder. The Vatican's fiat is clear. Would-be suicides, take heed: you'll plunge straight to hell's fiery depths should you foil God's plan by taking yourself out of the game before the ninth inning. Yet neither label, of criminal nor sinner, daunts those intent on the act.

Leslie Farber, in *The Ways of the Will,* considered "the life of suicide," which he says "must not be seen as the situation or state of mind which leads to the act, but that situation in which the act-as-possibility, quite apart from whether it eventually occurs or not, has a life of its own." Suicide is a conscious act, despite the fact that it is considered or undertaken "when the balance of the mind is disturbed." For some women with PMS, life becomes a torturous existence in which the act-as-possibility haunts their thoughts.

Ursula Pappert, one of our patients, said she contemplated suicide. "It really scared me because it seemed at that point it was beginning to get more control of me. Luckily that happened just before I went to the clinic for the first time. PMS is such a severe up and down, and it doesn't just last for an hour or something, it lasts for days. You get to the point where you can't take it anymore, and you really start feeling guilty about your family and everything. 'I must be an awfully terrible person, and I think they'd be better off if I weren't around.' I can understand how people can contemplate or even try it. I never tried it but I thought about it just before I got diagnosed at the clinic."

Cesare Pavese observed that "no one ever lacks a good reason for suicide;" women with extremely severe cases of premenstrual syndrome of long duration usually have more than one. Their pain is magnified by the frustration and impotence of not understanding what is causing their illness and failing to find a treatment for it. Most women with PMS who have reached for a razor blade or a bottle of pills have done so because they were weary of the chronic illness, weary of being told by their families they were hypochondriacs or crazy, weary of being told by physicians that nothing was wrong with them or that a hysterectomy would fix it all — but it didn't. An overwhelming, all-encompassing sense of alienation, loneliness, and worthlessness, bred of ignorance and misunderstanding, cloaks them in a cocoon of despair that eventually becomes impossible for others to penetrate. They want relief of the most permanent kind.

Suicidal depression, which A. Alvarez calls "a kind of spiritual winter, frozen, sterile, unmoving" appears as a recurring theme in the poetry and fiction of Sylvia Plath. For the last twenty years, Plath has been the woman writer most identified with suicide and depression. She wrote of and from her own experiences. Obsessed with the memory of her father who killed himself when she was eight, she attempted suicide three times, succeeding on the fourth try although from the cues she left behind she apparently intended to fail yet again. Throughout her poetry and the autobiographical novel, *The Bell Jar,* the theme of suicide resonates. The heroine of *The Bell Jar* weeps at her father's grave just before she holes up in a cellar and swallows fifty sleeping pills. An introductory note Plath wrote to *Daddy* before a reading of the poem on the BBC said the poem's narrator "has to act out the awful little allegory once over before she is free of it." In *Daddy,* Plath rails:

> "At twenty I tried to die
> And get back, back, back to you.
> I thought even the bones would do."

From *Lady Lazarus:*

> "I have done it again.
> One year in every ten
> I manage it...
> A sort of walking miracle...
> I am only thirty.
> And like the cat I have nine times to die.
> This is Number Three..."

Her obsession with purity, blood images, and death are also given major expression in her poetry. In *The Munich Mannequins,* she wrote, "Perfection is terrible. It cannot have children." In *Tulips,* the poet is ill and in the hospital, the flowers brought as a gift "are too red in the first place, they hurt me," and the smiling faces of her husband and children in a family photograph "catch on to my skin, little smiling hooks... I am a nun now, I have never been so pure." She wants to flee from the blood (the red tulips), the pain and the entanglements of close relationships into death. In *Fever 103* she wrote,

> "I am too pure for you or anyone.
> Your body
> Hurts me as the world hurts God."

A. Alvarez writes in *The Savage God* that Plath, "spoke of suicide with a wry detachment, and without any mention of the suffering or drama of the act... She seemed to view death as a physical challenge she had, once again, overcome. It was an experience of much the same quality as mastering a bolting horse... Suicide, in short, was not a swoon into death, an attempt 'to cease upon the midnight with no pain,' it was something to be felt in the nerve ends and fought against, an initiation rite qualifying her for a life of her own.''

Plath committed suicide after a difficult two-year period in which she had given birth to a daughter, suffered a miscarriage, had been hospitalized with appendicitis, gave birth to a son, and separated from her husband. After failing to kill herself in a car accident in late 1961, she tried again and succeeded on a frigid Monday morning in February, 1962. Depression, illness, and the starkness of winter, combined with the demands of two small children, were too much for her; she turned on the gas oven one morning but apparently thought she'd be found and saved because she had made an appointment with a new au pair girl for 9 A.M. that day and had left a note with her physician's name and number. Alvarez, then the poetry editor of *The Observer* of London, wrote: ''She lay down in front of the gas oven almost hopefully, almost with relief, as though she were saying, 'Perhaps this will set me free.' In part, I suppose, it was a 'cry for help' which fatally misfired. But it was also a last desperate attempt to exorcise the death she had summed up in her poems... when she and her husband separated, however mutual the arrangement, she again went through the same piercing grief and bereavement she had felt as a child when her father, by his death, seemed to abandon her.''

Despite the inexorable tie of depression, a women's disease, with suicide, women account for only slightly more than twenty-five percent of the suicides in this country each year, according to the U.S. Census Bureau, or about seven thousand of the twenty-seven thousand total. Researchers explain the discrepancy by noting that women are more likely to attempt suicide than men, but they succeed less often. The classic study, *Suicide and Attempted Suicide,* by Erwin Stengel in 1969 noted that ''the number of suicide attempts is six to ten times that of suicides;'' most data indicate that the ratio of men to women who attempt suicide is almost exactly the reverse of the ratio of men to women who complete suicide. Researchers also report that more women attempt suicide during the premenstrual phase than at other times in their cycle. Some of these attempts are made by women with premenstrual syndrome.

About ten percent of our patients have made a suicide attempt, and most of these women have made multiple attempts. About twenty percent of our patients, especially those who have PMS and a clinical depression, say they have had suicidal thoughts. Of the women who have PMS but do not have a pervasive clinical depression, some develop a profound depression on the second, third, fourth, or fifth day before their period; this is when the suicidal thoughts or attempts occur. These symptoms usually disappear after the period starts. But women who have PMS and a depression may have suicidal thoughts at any time during the month because they are suffering from two disorders.

Most common are the episodes of suicidal thoughts. Tracy Stevens, a mother of two, suffered from a postpartum depression so severe that she planned her entire life around the week and a half that she felt well. The rest of the time she spent in her room. She says she had planned her suicide in her mind. She didn't try to kill herself, although she desperately wanted to die, because "I couldn't leave my kids." The closest she came was just before she found out about the clinic, when she threw a glass against a kitchen cabinet and screamed at her husband, "You're not helping me. I need help!" Stephanie Lansing, twenty-four, also had severe depressions that eventually led to suicidal thoughts. "I talked a lot about not wanting to live," she said. "I just got so tired trying to get up the energy during my two good weeks to feel good enough to make it through the two bad weeks." Now symptom-free on progesterone therapy, she says, "When I think back on it, I just can't believe it."

Lynn Rousseau, the mother of three, also found she couldn't go through with suicide: "The big pain for me was the threat of losing this beautiful little family of mine. I never calculated how to do it or the cleanest way to go. I just thought about my car going off the mountainside. I know the embarrassment that comes from a suicide in the family. I would have chosen a way that looked like an accident. My death wish wasn't all selfish; I would have done it to prevent my family from living through this hell."

Thoughts of suicide and actual attempts have a complicated effect on the family. The murder of oneself is the ultimate violence, wreaked not only on the victim but on those closest to her. As Boris Pasternak wrote in *An Essay in Autobiography:* "...we have no conception of the inner torture which precedes suicide." A person "who decides to commit suicide puts a full stop to his being, he turns his back on his past, he declares himself a bankrupt and his memories to be unreal." But as Rollo May pointed out in *Power and Innocence,* when he writes of a patient, Priscilla, who remarked that a man she knew would not have committed suicide if "one person had known him" ... "I believe she was saying that this man had no person to whom he could open himself up, no one who was interested enough in him to listen, to pay attention to him.... he lacked someone who had compassion for him, a compassion which would be the basis of his self-esteem. If he had had such a person, he would have counted himself too valuable to wipe out."

At the same time that suicide and thoughts of suicide are a violence against the family, they can be a desperate cry for help and the recognition that might salvage self-esteem. The husband of thirty-seven-year-old Diana Marshall, who threatened to kill herself regularly, says, "She was angry, would cry incessantly, was shattered and debilitated. She'd run upstairs and lie on our bed, crying and talking about suicide. I'd tell her how much the children and I needed her. Sometimes, especially at the beginning, I thought that her threats were serious. But I'd been through it so many times — twelve times a year for ten years — and she always made it. I'd grit my teeth and bite my knuckles and say to myself, 'Here we go again.' I knew that nothing I said or did would improve the situation."

Maria Mancini, after suffering for ten years, started hoarding her painkillers and antidepressants prescribed for migraines and depression. Her parents, sisters, brother, and husband thought she was suicidal. "And I was. But I would never have committed suicide because I couldn't have left my two children. Yet death wasn't an enemy to me anymore. I think there are a lot more things worse than death. I think my brother [a physician] felt I needed to be committed. My parents didn't want to do that. My mother kept me at her house and put the medications away. She was afraid I would overdose."

When the trauma of premenstrual syndrome becomes too much for some women to handle, they actually try to take their own life. Fausta Martin, thirty-nine, married, two children, attempted suicide in the fall of 1977. "I swallowed a bottle of Valium about nine o'clock, after I had been drinking all evening. It was the culmination of two weeks of suicidal thoughts. I had been thinking about using razor blades, or crashing the car into a tree. I'd had suicidal thoughts for about two years, during those two weeks out of the month. But I was a fighter. I fought my symptoms all the way. I made myself go out no matter how difficult it was, because it was better than the isolated depression of staying home alone. By the fall of 1977 I had had enough. I just gave up. I felt that my husband and my children would be better off without me. I couldn't see getting better, and I couldn't live a nightmare anymore. By that time I didn't even have a two-week grace period. The two weeks were so terrible that the months just ran into each other.''

Her husband was downstairs. Her two children were asleep. "I just couldn't live like that anymore. I'd fought it for so long. I'd tried so many different things and there wasn't a cure. I felt as if I had done everything that I could have done. My husband had stopped loving me and given up. I can't say that I blame him. I woke up the next morning and told my husband what I had done. I was lucky that I woke up. The Valium that I took was only two milligrams per tablet, although I didn't know that when I swallowed them. My husband took me to the emergency room. They didn't pump my stomach, but they kept me in the hospital for three days. My husband was shocked and angry. It was the last straw. His patience had run out. I vaguely remembered while I was driving around in my car that afternoon that he was supposed to go to a conference on the West Coast that evening. But I didn't get back until the early evening, so he missed his conference. I suppose I did it deliberately.'' Her children were four and seven at the time; she never told them about the incident.

Her husband Jack remembers the episode started after ''we had had an enormous battle. I was so angry and furious that I didn't care what she did. She told me that she was going to the car to commit suicide, and I told her to go ahead and do it. When she came back, I told myself that I knew she would. She came upstairs, and I had no idea of what she'd done until she told me the next morning. I called poison control and brought her to the hospital, but I was angry that she was destroying the family and my life. I felt like I wanted someone else to look after her for a while. I'd know that I had to take care of her, but I was still angry.''

In perhaps the most extreme case we have encountered, one woman, Phyllis Schwartz, was forced to sign away the custody of her children after she made a suicide attempt. (She is now involved in a court battle

for their return). Schwartz says she took an overdose of many medica
tions after "a hellish day and night in which I was out of control. I ha
overdosed on not one bottle of pills, but a multiple of all my medica
tions. My heart stopped and my breathing stopped. I didn't call fo
anyone, they found me unconscious. But I know now that it will neve
happen to me again."

The extreme symptoms that push some women to the very brink o
death are rare, but as these interviews reveal they are a real part of som
women's lives. Most women with PMS choose a troublesome life ove
death, even though, as the Russian poet Mayakovsky wrote:

> "In this life it is not difficult to die
> It is more difficult to live."

Maybe, as Dorothy Parker told us in *Resumé,* suicide is really mor
trouble than it's worth:

> "Guns aren't lawful;
> Nooses give;
> Gas smells awful;
> You might as well live."

SECTION IV / *Female Complaints*

Chapter 13

> *"Women are growing honester, braver,*
> *stronger, more healthful and skillful*
> *and able and free..."*
>
> Charlotte Perkins Gilman, **Woman and Economics**

The Pill

Jogging and oral contraceptives probably represent the most common daily, shared experience of American women. Nearly forty million of them have taken oral contraceptives at some point in their life; nine million take them now. Despite a plethora of minor side effects and the potential for major ones, women continue to pop the Pill as acceptingly as they lace up their Nikes and jog around the park. They value the result even if it's accompanied by fluid retention or a case of shin splints. The Pill fulfills its promise: it's the safest form of contraception — about 99.5 percent effective. For three decades it has held sway as the magic bullet, a guarantee against unwanted pregnancy and a key to unprecedented sexual freedom. Some women with PMS — especially those whose symptoms started early and who have less severe cases — may find that they are more interested in sex during the premenstrual phase, contradicting research studies that report that most women have a decreased interest in sex just prior to menstruation. Many women trace the onset of PMS to their taking of oral contraceptives, and the Pill generally exacerbates all premenstrual symptoms, particularly weight gain, fluid retention, depression, and headaches. About sixty percent of our patients have taken the Pill at some time; only about ten percent currently use oral contraceptives.

Martine Hudson began taking the Pill one month before her wedding in 1970 and that triggered her premenstrual symptoms. "I became irritable and depressed. My parents and then-fiance became worried about me. On our way to our honeymoon I told my husband I wanted to come home," she remembers. "For the first six months I bled every day. I had constant migraines and depression which I didn't tell anybody about, as well as strange hair growth, swollen breasts. I told my doctor about the symptoms and she put me on *two* birth control pills a day. My symptoms just went crazy. I then told her that I was very depressed and didn't know why, that I cried all day. The bleeding had stopped though. She told me then that all those symptoms were because of the birth control pills. She said she hadn't told me this before so I wouldn't imagine symptoms that weren't there." Recalling the episode, Hudson paused and emphasized: "I was *very* angry. If I had known what to look for, I would have been off those pills so fast. It took three months after stopping the pill for the symptoms to subside. But some of them didn't. It was then that I noticed a cyclical pattern to it all. I noticed weepiness and moods premenstrually. Then I became pregnant with my first daughter." What followed was a difficult pregnancy, marked by migraine, bloating, weight gain, outbursts, and ten years of classic and devastating premenstrual syndrome.

Another patient, Carmen Estes also had an immediate reaction. "There were definite symptoms from the first month I was married and started on the birth control pill: fatigue, weight gain, and immediate vision change. I required glasses and had a sense that it wasn't so much blurring as distortion in space. I gained fifteen pounds in one month. As a teenager, I had no acne, but from the time I took the birth control pill on, my face was extremely broken out. My doctor was smart enough to say that I never should have been put on the pill. After getting off the pill, I was still in a state of imbalance." Later Estes had toxemia with pregnancy, severe postpartum depression, and half a dozen other premenstrual complaints.

The Hormone Reaction

Hormones are the villains of these stories. The Pill prevents pregnancy by changing the body's hormonal balance. There are two types of oral contraceptives available: the "combined" estrogen-progestogen pill and the progestogen-only, or mini-pill. Until recently there was a third, called the "sequential" pill. Sequential contraceptives involved taking estrogen only pills for the first fifteen days of the cycle, then estrogen-progestogen pills for the remaining five days. Sequential were removed from the market because they were unreliable and became associated with an increased risk of endometrial cancer.

The combined pill, the more popular type, contains an estrogen and a progestogen analog of testosterone — a substance with progestational properties. Two types of estrogens, which are very similar, are used, one of which is more potent than the other. Many different types of progestogens are used; each have slightly different effects on the other hormones in the body. Some progestogens antagonize the effects of estrogen and lead to the unpleasant side effects of breast swelling and tenderness; weight gain, fluid retention, even acne and headaches. When the Pill was first developed in 1951 it contained only progestogen; estrogen was thought to be carcinogenic. But the pure progestogen pill resulted in spotting — bleeding between menstruation — so estrogen was added. But the pharmaceutical makers overdid it. Estrogen was added so copiously that it was later found to be five times as much as needed, up to 100 micrograms in some brands. Today the pill contains between 20 and 30 micrograms of estrogen; in rare cases it is as high as 50 micrograms. The dosage was drastically slashed to alleviate the side effects caused by the large amounts of estrogen and as a safety measure because of fears that estrogen would lead to cervical, endometrial, or ovarian cancer. Despite the fact that estrogen has not been found to cause these cancers, the drug companies are continuing to research methods of producing a pill with still less estrogen.

The brand of combined pill and the amount of estrogen needed varies with the individual. Most gynecologists prefer to start a woman on a low dosage and scale upward if needed, to lessen possible side effects. If the dosage is too low, spotting will occur because the amount of estrogen is not sufficient to support the endometrial lining of the uterus. There's also a chance that ovulation will not be suppressed and pregnancy could occur. But if the dose is too high, it is more difficult to cut down because spotting will result once the uterus — which has come to rely on more estrogen than normal to bolster the endometrium — finds that the extra support is suddenly withdrawn. High amounts of estrogen also increase the risk of stroke or heart attacks. The combined pill is sold under a spectrum of brand names including Brevicon, Demulen, Enovid, Lo/Ovral, Loestrin, Modicon, Norinyl, Norlestrin, Ortho-Novum, Ovral, Ovulen, and Zorane. These are usually taken in cycles of three weeks on and one week off, beginning typically on the fifth day of the menstrual cycle. For those who have trouble adhering to this schedule, there is a brand that can be taken every day; the one week off is represented by seven hormone-less pills.

The progestogen-only or mini-pill, sold under the brand names Micronor and Ovrette, is less reliable than the combined pill because it does not prevent ovulation. Instead, it interferes with the permeability of the cervical mucus to sperm, preventing the sperm from reaching the egg, and by disturbing the growth of the endometrium, so that implantation of a fertilized egg cannot take place. The mini-pill is recommended for women who cannot tolerate the side effects of estrogen. Also, it's taken every day so its regimen is easier to follow. Nonetheless, women on the mini-pill may notice increased, frequently heavy spotting because progestogens halt the growth of the endometrium so it is constantly sloughing off. Progestogens also alter the motility of the Fallopian tubes with the result of an increased risk of ectopic, or tubal, pregnancies.

The primary function of the combined pill is to prevent ovulation. Initially, the combined estrogen-progestogen prevents the release of FSH by the hypothalamus-pituitary. Consequently, the egg follicles are not stimulated and no egg is produced. Menstruation, however, occurs because the estrogen-progestogen pill is stimulating endometrial growth and withdrawal. When the pill is stopped for one week, the growth of the endometrium halts and it sloughs off. This bleeding is commonly referred to as a "false period," because the bleeding occurs but for the wrong reasons. The mini-pill does not interfere with the release of FSH, nor with the FSH and LH surge that produces the release of the egg from the ovary. Thus, the body remains ready for fertilization. But the mini-pill thickens the cervical mucus, which then traps the sperm and prevents fertilization. Because ovulation does occur, there is a much greater risk of getting pregnant. In addition, the mini-pill carries greater risk of ectopic, or tubal, pregnancies, and of high blood pressure and increased blood clotting.

The Pill As Protector

Since its development thirty years ago, the Pill and its users have been carefully scrutinized because the drug was feared to be factor in endometrial, cervical, and ovarian cancers. However, over the past five years, studies have shown that the Pill, especially the combined pill, actually protects women from an array of disorders, including benign breast disease, ovarian cysts, iron deficiency anemia, pelvic inflammatory disease, and tubal pregnancies, and may also reduce the risk of rheumatoid arthritis, endometrial and ovarian cancer. Dr. Howard Ory of the Center for Disease Control in Atlanta, says the Pill saves women fifty thousand hospitalizations a year for these diseases.

The persistent problems that remain with the Pill of all types are an increased risk of developing blood clotting disorders which can lead to a stroke, and a suspicion that it can cause liver disease and tumors. Estrogen causes the walls of blood veins to dilate, which decreases blood flow. It also interferes with the normal clotting mechanism by making the blood platelets stickier, so that more and larger clots appear. This increased tendency toward clots may provoke heart attacks. But recent studies have shown that fatal clots, in women who are otherwise not predisposed to them, occur in about three out of one hundred thousand women taking the Pill. This incidence is minimal when compared with pregnancy and delivery mortality rates of twenty-five per one hundred thousand women. In women over thirty-five years of age, the Pill may lead to circulatory disorders; women who smoke should not use the Pill at all since it increases their risk of circulatory and blood clotting problems to dangerous levels.

While the reduced dosages of estrogen in the Pill may ease its side effects in many women, the Pill's triggering effect on women predisposed to premenstrual syndrome remains unchanged. In fact, we're likely to see a larger PMS population because of the Pill. Its popularity as a tool to control irregular and painful menstruation led gynecologists to prescribe it for large numbers of adolescent girls, beginning in the 1960s and continuing through the present. The exposure of these girls to the Pill at a much earlier age than their mothers or older sisters means they will have been on the Pill for more years by the time they move into their twenties and thirties and decide to stop taking it and start families. This group of women, then, are at extremely high risk to develop PMS. It is a large group, representing the tail end of the postwar baby boom. We expect that increased numbers of these women will develop PMS either as a reaction to the Pill itself or later, after a subsequent pregnancy, hysterectomy, or tubal ligation. Instead of demand for PMS treatment declining as more is known about it and more physicians treat it, the demand may actually climb because the pool of women at risk will be larger.

Chapter 14

> *"That she bear children is not a woman's significance.*
> *But that she bear herself,*
> *That is her supreme and risky fate."*
>
> D.H. Lawrence, Women in Love

Pregnancy

Pregnancy imbues many women with a serenity of sorts, a sensation of physical well-being that is undoubtedly the source of the inner radiance and knowing glow that so many mothers-to-be are said to possess. Their birth experience meshes with that described by Sandra McPherson in her poem, *Pregnancy:*

> "It is the best thing.
> I should always like to be pregnant..."

Most of our patients who have been pregnant say they felt well, wonderful, terrific, even euphoric then. That's not surprising, since pregnancy is probably the only time they've received the most effective therapy for premenstrual syndrome — progesterone, in large doses. During the last two trimesters of pregnancy, a woman's body produces enormous amounts of progesterone to sustain the fetus. The word progesterone means just that: pro gestation, to aid pregnancy. For the vast majority of the women we see, pregnancy was the only time in their lives that they ever felt well. (Eighty percent of our patients are mothers.) They're not alone. A study by Drs. Raymond Greene and Katharina Dalton in 1953 noted that of fifty-nine women with PMS, ninety-three percent were symptom-free during the middle and last trimester of pregnancy and sixty-two percent remarked on their improved health and increased energy.

Women with severe premenstrual syndrome whose daily lives have been disrupted for one to three weeks a month for several years often choose pregnancy over PMS. One of our patients said she and her husband had planned to have four children but ended up having eight because the only time that she was comfortable and that her relationship with her husband was positive was when she was pregnant. Luckily they could afford a large family. No one is advocating that women should be or like to be kept barefoot and pregnant; but some women in extreme pain — physical or psychological — have developed a kind of primitive self-help program, opting to be bound to a large brood rather than trapped by PMS.

Some women with PMS have a difficult time in the first trimester when progesterone levels are still relatively low, but they begin to feel fine — often better than fine — in the second and third trimesters. About thirty percent of our patients have a history of miscarriages or threatened abortion during the first trimester. Some physicians suggest that's because of a deficiency of progesterone during the luteal phase of the menstrual cycle. A luteal phase deficiency would mean that these women don't have enough progesterone in their systems to sustain pregnancy. Many gynecologists treat women with a history of miscarriages in the first trimester because of a luteal phase deficiency with progesterone during the luteal phase, 25 to 50 milligrams twice a day.

Toxemia in Pregnancy

For some women pregnancy is not a pleasant experience; it can even be life-threatening to mother and child. Instead of having a sense of well-being or euphoria, they suffer from toxemia, a condition marked by severe hypertension, swelling of the ankles, feet, hands and face, dizziness and spots in front of the eyes, and dangerously high weight gain. The condition affects a surprisingly large number of women, about ten to fifteen percent of all pregnant women, particularly those in lower income groups, teenagers, and older women undergoing their first pregnancy. Severe toxemia can lead to convulsions or stroke, may cause liver or kidney damage, and occasionally requires the abortion of the fetus to save the life of the mother. Toxemia accounts for twenty percent of all maternal deaths in this country. The cause of the disorder is unknown but because it disappears after delivery some researchers suggest that the placenta is somehow involved in the massive retention of salt and water that leads to the physical signs of this condition. About ninety-six percent of the women who suffer toxemia in pregnancy will subsequently develop PMS.

Difficult births are common for women who experience toxemia during pregnancy. Whether this has anything to do with the premenstrual syndrome, however, is problematic. We know that most women with PMS or women who later develop PMS do not endure toxemic pregnancies. Rather they may feel well or even wonderful during their pregnancies, especially during the second and third trimesters. But we know from our own practice and from reports of case histories of other physicians that some women who have been treated for PMS experienced some kind of difficulty during the delivery of their babies. Not enough data is available to determine if this is a rare, infrequent, or common occurrence. It is not surprising, however, to encounter women with PMS who have had other reproductive-related health problems.

Several of our patients who have had abortions say that PMS symptoms started after the abortion. But we haven't seen enough patients with these experiences to determine if they have the same or different patterns from women who have never conceived or women who have carried a fetus to term. And some women develop PMS after a pregnancy; these women usually find that the symptoms worsen after each subsequent pregnancy.

It is extremely rare for a women to experience premenstrual symptoms during a pregnancy, but Mary Waters, a woman treated by a colleague in a Western state, says her problems developed with her third and last pregnancy four years ago. "I started the symptoms even before I knew I was pregnant; it lasted during the first three months of the term." The symptoms disappeared and then reappeared with great intensity about six months after the delivery of the baby. Her problems have been eliminated with progesterone therapy, diet changes, and Vitamin B_6.

Multiple pregnancies and the incidence of toxemia in pregnancy sharply increase the probability that a woman will develop premenstrual syndrome.

Chapter 15

> *There is a Languor of the Life*
> *More imminent than Pain*
> *'Tis Pain's Successor — When the Soul*
> *Has suffered all it can —*
>
> Emily Dickinson

Post-Partum Depression

Like nuggets of coal meanly tucked into a child's Christmas stocking, postpartum depression is an anti-climax. After months of excited anticipation of the most awesome mystery of life, birth, the baby blues arrive as an uninvited guest. It swaddles some mothers in a draining gloom, a psychological barrier to their enjoyment of the baby. Struggling to break out of the smothering gauze, they cry and rage, their frustration rises. Matty Quest, the protagonist of Doris Lessing's novel, *A Proper Marriage,* waddled through a discomfiting pregnancy and unexpectedly painful delivery of her first child, Caroline, only to find that her state of mind grows worse not better. At one point she tells the baby: "My poor unfortunate brat, what had you done to deserve a mother like me? ... You bore me to extinction, and that's the truth of it, and no doubt I bore you... you and I are just victims, my poor child, you can't help it, I can't help it, my mother couldn't help it, and her mother..." For some women, the depression is apocalyptic, a slap in the face from God; it shatters their daily existence, leading to rejection of the baby and withdrawal from family and society. In extreme cases, it may lead to suicidal thoughts or suicide attempts.

Twenty to forty percent of our patients have experienced postpartum depression, usually for long periods of seven to twelve months. (These are separate from the thirty percent of our patients who exhibit both a current depression as well as PMS.) It apparently accelerates or exacerbates the development of premenstrual syndrome or is part of the mechanism that produces PMS. Identifying this condition is not always easy; depression is a common disorder in women and depression is a symptom of premenstrual syndrome. A true postpartum depression is just what it sounds like: a woman becomes pregnant, delivers, and develops a depression that continues for a length of time. Some physicians say any depressed state that runs for at least two weeks qualifies; others require a longer episode before they'll make the diagnosis.

As one of our patients, Fran Harris, recalls: "It's just a very strong depression. You say to yourself, 'I should be happy. I have this beautiful brand new baby.' But you're not, you're just not happy. You're always rationalizing why you feel this way. You say to yourself, 'I haven't had much sleep lately because of the baby.' But I think that most people are just trying to find a reason why they're just sitting there and crying. You get to be like a recluse. You don't want to go out." After the birth of her second child, her depression was severe. "With the baby, I stayed in the house a lot. It was beautiful then, July. There was no good reason to stay in the house, but I stayed in the house a lot. I would cry, sit in the chair and cry. I felt the depression right after the birth of the child. I remember feeling bad in the hospital. I don't think a lot of women understand it and I know a lot of husbands don't. Mine was really skeptical."

Shirley deVereaux, forty-seven, has five children, thirteen to twenty-five, and had postpartum depression "with every child. It was worse with the second and third, probably because I had them in such rapid succession. I was bogged down, and more or less on my own. At that time my mother was still having children and was sickly, and I had two of hers all the time, so I had five little ones."

Agoraphobia and Other Fears

Lee Arnold went through "a really severe postpartum depression after the birth of my daughter. I think it was longer than usual from other women I've talked to. It seems that we all develop these awful depressions. Mine was so bad that I was starting to develop a fear of going out of the house, agoraphobia. Just getting on clothes and getting the baby dressed and getting in the car and going to the store was just too much trouble to imagine. I didn't blame it on anyone, I just thought it was me. I thought that I had to get myself out of this. I did notice after about two or three months that it was cyclical. I just wanted to lie in bed and not even get up on those days before my period. I think that's how I probably kept myself from becoming very angry."

Jackie Weber, the mother of three, came close to rejecting her baby completely. After the birth of her first child, "my husband recalls how surprised he was at the hospital that I was not drawn to this new little baby. He expected this motherly instinct to flow because it always had in his mother. She has eight children. I didn't have any idea that he saw this in me. I didn't have a real interest in the baby. I wanted to breast feed but that wasn't going well. The baby cried all the time and I thought that was normal. This is what motherhood is all about. The struggle began almost immediately. I was very nervous but, because of the expectations of everyone, I pretended that I was very happy about the whole thing and faked my way through it all as it turned out. I felt desperate. I didn't care, I was not drawn to the baby. I had really wanted the baby and I was overjoyed when I found out I was pregnant, and it was a boy and we wanted a boy. But I felt no emotional commitment. I was nervous anyway and shaky. I cried a lot. The baby allowed me no sleep and because the baby was so demanding I didn't feel well. I remember inwardly feeling like my life had ended, but I did not project that on the surface." She added, "My best friend had a baby the same month and we used to go everywhere together. Her little baby never cried and she felt so well. I remember trying to be lighthearted like her. She was calm, I wasn't. Her baby slept, mine cried."

After the birth of her second child, Weber suffered from postpartum depression for two years and was treated with Tofranil. "I responded well for five days and then it didn't work anymore." After her third delivery, the postpartum depression was severe but her doctor refused to prescribe Tofranil when she asked for it because he said it was addictive. After this third birth, "I suffered three weeks out each month. I was severely depressed. I felt like I was going to die. I was so depressed, so angry. And there was no way I could hide these feelings any longer, the way I did with the first two deliveries. I would often make excuses and stay home from church meetings and social events, or I'd go late or duck out early so I wouldn't erupt. I thought I was mentally ill. I screamed at the children, felt like throwing them out a window, wanted to divorce my husband, wanted to throw things, books, anything, across the room." After seeing dozens of doctors in three different cities in which they lived, she saw a physician who diagnosed her properly as having PMS. But his treatment was to do a hysterectomy followed by monthly estrogen implants, a painful process.

Psychiatric Problems Encountered

Postpartum depression is an extremely common disorder. The psychological or physiological stress of childbirth precipitates not only postpartum depression but other psychiatric problems as well. The ancient healers, Celsus, Galen, and Soranus, all recorded cases of postpartum psychosis. An English study reported that sixty-six percent of a random sample of women who delivered at one hospital later suffered from postpartum depression at least briefly. And many studies show that women are more likely to be admitted to a psychiatric hospital after delivery than at other times in their lives. A study of seventy-one women over seventeen years with post-delivery psychiatric admissions revealed that forty percent of the cases began within a week of delivery.

Another research project involving seven women with postpartum depression evidenced the link with the premenstrual syndrome. Typically, it noted, women suffer from a relatively mild postpartum depression in the thirties or late twenties, with an average age of onset of thirty. "Emotional stress or an infective illness may have coincided with postpartum time. She appears to recover but then relapses. Then for years she suffers from recurrent phases of depression, irritability, tension, with phobias, obsessive fears, or hypochondria. The severity of her symptoms is related to the menstrual cycle, usually the premenstrual phase. Her moodiness, unpredictability, and loss of temper are reacted to by the children and the husband, the family atmosphere becomes clouded and unstable, and the family ceases to function as a unified group." It's a profile that fits many of our patients.

After Andrea Neubecker's daughter was born, she was mildly depressed, with "no drastic emotional changes. Things started to get to the point where I knew they were wrong about five years later." Then, she said, each month she experienced "times of very unusual fatigue, a slight roller coaster effect. I'd be worn out by 7 P.M., I'd be laid out on the couch. Tests showed nothing. We moved that year, and I think that the stress and the change and the move probably aggravated it. It really became disabling by 1980. Things were really getting out of control as far as crying and feeling that I couldn't keep up with things, worthlessness. Almost everything was directed at myself, inward. I don't think other than a very rare occasion when I'd let it it out on my husband. I don't think I ever acted out toward the children. It was always inward. I avoided contact with people. You're not sure of yourself so you don't want to be around other people."

Dr. Katharina Dalton investigated postpartum depression prospectively by focusing on a group of women without PMS and following them through pregnancy and afterward. She found that of the women who experienced postpartum depression, about seventy-six percent subsequently developed PMS. Unfortunately, most of the studies in this area have not distinguished women with postpartum depression who have never had a previous depressive episode from women who have had one or many depressions prior to the pregnancy. What seems to happens is this: women with postpartum depression are depressed steadily all month-long for a period of time; then they begin to feel better; then they get worse; then better and then worse, and on and on, creating a cycle. The postpartum depression and additional symptoms, like breast swelling and tenderness, eventually become confined to the premenstrual phase, resulting in PMS.

Grace Henson fits this cycle-creation pattern. Henson, a stockbroker with four children, remembers: "After the last pregnancy (twins) I went through a very bad baby blues, and it just didn't seem that I came out of it. Once my period started, my first period was an ovulatory period, I just hemorrhaged and was rushed back to the hospital. After that, I'd be okay for a couple of weeks and then I'd slip back into it. I'd just be crying all the time. Naturally this especially affected the children. I never got to the point of taking it out on them or being overly angry with them. I took it out more on my husband. We fought constantly. Finally it got very difficult in April. But again my case is a little different. Twin births are extremely difficult for parents, especially when you have other children. To this day, they don't sleep through the night. When you have babies up all night long, and you're not getting any sleep on top of everything else that's going on, well, I'm just glad I didn't find a cliff and jump off it. As far as relating to the family, I just felt that nobody understood me, and that I couldn't understand myself, so I started counseling about two months after the baby was born. I have kept that up because I found that it was doing a terrific amount of good."

The cause of postpartum depression isn't known, but there are many theories. Some researchers have suggested that an imbalance between the relative levels of estrogens and progesterone in the period immediately following delivery is the trigger; others say there may be a kind of rebound effect — an overproduction of hormones — following the loss of the placenta that the body can't handle. The view espoused by Dr. Dalton is based on a feast-and-famine analogy. The hormonal swings of the menstrual cycle are infinitesimal compared with the massive increase in placental steroid hormones, including progesterone, during pregnancy and the abrupt deprivation of these hormones following delivery. This zenith/nadir effect calls for a remarkable adjustment on the part of the woman. This dramatic shift in hormone levels results in many women experiencing what's tantamount to an addict going cold turkey: feeling the euphoric glow in late pregnancy, probably caused by the huge amounts of progesterone in the bloodstream, followed by the progesterone deprivation and depths of depression.

A forty-five-year-old mother of six children, Marty Eisner, experienced the depths of postpartum depression after the birth of each child. She recalls, ''When I was pregnant, it was the only time in my whole life that I really felt terrific. Now I know that this is the way normal people feel all the time.''

Progesterone is not a treatment for depression but it may help postpartum depression. Interestingly, our patients who have had postpartum depression usually require more progesterone to alleviate their symptoms than women who haven't had the baby blues.

Chapter 16

"Chaste to her husband, frank to all beside,
A teeming mistress, but a barren bride."

Alexander Pope, **Moral Essays**

Sterilization

After the birth of her third child, and at the suggestion of her gynecologist, thirty-six-year-old Marlene Swift underwent a sterilization procedure known as a tubal ligation. "It seemed to make a lot of sense at the time," Swift says. "My husband and I weren't planning to have any more children and my physician recommended it as a permanent, safe, easy method of birth control." Tubal ligations involve the severing of the Fallopian tubes so an egg cannot reach the uterus. Unlike its sister procedure, hysterectomy, tubal ligation usually does not affect the ovaries, halt the production of progesterone and estrogen, or stop menstruation. What Swift was soon to discover is that there are many complications from this "safe, easy" procedure that about seven hundred thousand American women undergo each year. But painful menstruation and pelvic inflammation, or heavy and prolonged bleeding are frequent results. For some women, like Marlene Swift, premenstrual syndrome is another. About twenty percent of our patients have had tubal ligations; in almost every case the procedure seemed to trigger PMS or a worsening of pre-existing PMS.

Paula Thompson had a tubal ligation one month after the youngest of her two children was born. She, like many of our patients, found an array of problems soon developed, including irritability and temper tantrums, postpartum depression, suicidal thoughts, and some minor scuffles with her husband and children. The premenstrual symptoms continued to worsen until she began progesterone treatment and lifestyle changes; now she's symptom-free.

Eileen Alpert developed premenstrual syndrome at puberty. "After my second child was born four years ago, I started constant bleeding. I was given a D&C; that didn't stop it; I was given Provera. I also had my tubes tied. Right at that particular time I noticed there was a drastic change in me. It wasn't just minor, it was a complete change. An emotional change." Alpert was depressed, developed cyclical insomnia, acne, food cravings, colitis, and migraine headaches. All these complaints disappeared when she began treatment for PMS.

Hysterectomy is the surgical removal of the uterus and/or the removal of the ovaries; about six hundred fifty thousand women undergo hysterectomies in this country each year. It results in sterilization but good physicians do not perform this procedure merely as a permanent method of birth control. The most common reason for hysterectomy is to excise large, usually benign, fibroid tumors of the uterus that can cause severe menstrual bleeding, lead to anemia, and potentially to ovarian cancer. Fibroid tumors can reach the size of a ten- to twelve-week-old fetus, filling the pelvic cavity; three percent of women who develop fibroids die of ovarian cancer. In women under forty-five, surgeons now leave the ovaries intact unless there's irrevocable damage, such as a malignant tumor that doesn't respond to other therapy. Removing the ovaries induces early menopause and increases the threat of degenerative bone disease and heart disease. Estrogen replacement therapy is almost always prescribed for women following a hysterectomy, which in itself is risky; the use of estrogen increases the risk of endometrial cancer three to eight times. For these reasons, if one ovary is damaged or diseased, surgeons usually leave the other one in women who are still menstruating so they won't develop postmenopausal symptoms. Healthy ovaries may be removed with the uterus if a woman is near menopause, or if there is uterine cancer because cancer of the female reproductive organ may be hormone-stimulated.

Depression May Result

Another major postoperative complication of hysterectomy is depression. A study of more than seven hundred women who had undergone hysterectomy revealed that two and a half times as many psychiatric referrals were made for women who had had hysterectomies than those who hadn't: seven percent for the hysterectomy cases vs. three percent for the control group. The incidence of divorce and marital disruption after hysterectomy was also significantly higher than for the control group. Of the patients referred to a psychiatrist after the operation, eighty-five percent were suffering from depression, and sixty-six percent had also been referred to at least one other medical specialist for complaints ranging from nervousness to exhaustion, insomnia, and depression. Twenty-eight percent were admitted to a hospital for an overdose of drugs. Some of these diagnoses may have masked incidence of premenstrual syndrome.

About ten percent of our patients have undergone hysterectomies. Women who had premenstrual symptoms prior to the hysterectomy or tubal ligations usually experience a worsening of the PMS. Despite the fact that radical hysterectomy, the removal of the uterus and ovaries, induces menopause — and many women find that premenstrual syndrome symptoms end at menopause — some women who have had their ovaries removed continue to have cyclical symptoms. For a small number of women, the problems worsen. Dr. Katharina Dalton believes this is because their ovaries are no longer producing any progesterone. A typical pattern following hysterectomy is an end to the symptoms for six months to a year followed by a recurrence of premenstrual syndrome in a more severe form. A few women who say they did not have PMS prior to a hysterectomy trace the onset of their condition to the hysterectomy. Where cyclical symptoms continue or begin after this procedure, the timing tends to follow the pattern of the prior menstrual cycle. If the cycle was twenty-eight to thirty days prior to the hysterectomy, the PMS symptoms will recur every twenty-eight to thirty days. The most common cyclical symptoms following hysterectomy are headaches, depression, dizziness, fatigue, joint and muscle pain. We don't know why PMS occurs or worsens after a radical hysterectomy but it's probably tied to the mechanism for menstruation, the hypothalamus and pituitary. Some physicians recommend hysterectomies as a therapy for premenstrual syndrome and say their experience has shown that it relieves the symptoms; some theories about PMS say this might happen if the ovaries have been secreting a substance that produces the symptoms. In some women, hysterectomy produces no change in their symptoms at all.

More research needs to be undertaken into the function and effects of progesterone and estrogen, and the disposition and impact of hysterectomies in women with different symptoms and characteristics. The possibility that the sex hormones have functions beyond that of reproduction has not been fully explored; the predominance of premenstrual syndrome, however, could be an indication that the progesterone and estrogen do have more far-reaching functions than is now thought.

SECTION V / *Life Phases*

Chapter 17

"*Things she had never noticed much before
began to hurt her; home lights watched
from the evening sidewalks, an unknown
voice from an alley. She would stare at the
lights and listen to the voice, and something
inside her stiffened and waited. But the
lights would darken, the voice fall silent,
and though she waited, that was all. She
was afraid of these things that made her
suddenly wonder who she was, and what
she was going to be in the world, and why
she was standing at that minute, seeing a
light, or listening, or staring up into the
sky: alone. She was afraid, and there was
a queer tightness in her chest... Because
she could not break this tightness gathering
within her, she would hurry to do
something.*"

Carson McCullers, **The Member of the Wedding**

Adolescence

The tumult of adolescence is like being lost in a funhouse: the distortion of reality is brief but seemingly endless at the time; what's billed as a barrel of laughs is more typically a frustrating, frightening, panic-inducing run through a maze of booby traps and trick mirrors. When you're caught in that space and time, you just want out.

Teenage girls struggling to grow into their bodies and their emotions are perhaps those who suffer most from premenstrual syndrome. In most instances neither they nor their parents are able to distinguish a medically treatable problem as complex as PMS from the accepted traumas of adolescence. Extreme and bizarre behavior in teenagers that is neither socially acceptable nor part of any well-known illness has on a few occasions been diagnosed as a psychological disorder, periodic psychosis of puberty. We think that these cases are very likely premenstrual syndrome; the fact that an entirely new psychiatric category has been developed to describe it underscores the confusion about PMS in adolescents.

The forty or so teenagers we have treated have had severe cases; in a few instances they were brought in for evaluation because their mother or another relative also has premenstrual syndrome and was familiar with its pattern. As physicians and the public become educated about PMS, identifying it early will become easier. Puberty is one of the stages of life at which a significant percentage of women first experience the symptoms of PMS. Estimates of the incidence of the syndrome in adolescents vary from twenty to thirty percent of the teenagers who visit physicians for various complaints; few of these girls have been or are likely to be properly diagnosed and treated. One pediatrician in Boston, a patient of ours, says she has observed a great number of girls with PMS in her practice; since she's undergone the evaluation process herself she's been able to diagnose them and refer them for treatment.

A Loss of Identity

The crisis of adolescence, of course, is loss of identity as "the body changes its proportions radically, when genital puberty floods body and imagination with all manner of impulses, when intimacy with the other sex approaches and is, on occasion, forced on the young person, and when the immediate future confronts one with too many conflicting possibilities and choices," as Erik Erikson writes in *Identity Youth and Crisis*.

The sense of self that a girl may have gripped so confidently in childhood — I am me, my parents' child — seems to have evaporated without warning, like perfume in an unsealed flacon. Who am I? is the $64,000 question she poses. And she needs the answer fast, for "... in the social jungle of human existence there is no feeling of being alive without a sense of identity," Erikson says. No longer a child but not yet an adult, a teenager becomes frustrated and rebellious, poised for insolence or tears depending on which hormone surges first and fullest. It's a confusing phase, as voiced by Biff, in Arthur Miller's *Death of a Salesman:* "I just can't take hold, Mom. I can't take hold of some kind of life." For an adolescent girl, PMS intensifies the already formidable problems she faces in coming to terms with her emerging maturity, sexuality, sense of self, and relationship to family, authority, and peers.

Menstruation brings with it painful episodes of cramps to many teenagers, and irregular cycles to others. Those problems by and large are diagnosed and treated without much difficulty. But the presence of any or several of the symptoms of premenstrual syndrome can be far more crippling, physically and emotionally, than dysmenorrhea. PMS can even develop in a girl before menstruation begins. It sometimes takes hold at puberty, anytime from age eight to thirteen, but usually around eleven. Menarche, or the actual menstrual flow, may occur as much as two years later. In this age group, the syndrome is often marked by frequent, recurring attacks of asthma or epilepsy, striking just prior to menstruation or at menstruation. The attacks may occur at other times, as well, but are usually more frequent or more severe prior to menstruation. Girls whose episodes are usually well controlled with drugs may require more medication or find that it is less effective just prior to their period. Many of our patients, now in their twenties and thirties, whose asthma or epilepsy began in adolescence have been able to sharply reduce or discontinue their medications once they've been treated with progesterone. Anorexia nervosa may also appear in a teenager with premenstrual syndrome.

What parents usually fail to identify are the behavioral symptoms or the cyclicality of any symptoms, physical or psychological. If an otherwise well-behaved, normal girl periodically and regularly shows a marked change in mood or reaction a few days each month for several months at home or at school or both, and then reverts to her regular behavior, she may well have a mild form of premenstrual syndrome. It's more serious if she's rebellious or has difficulty concentrating, especially if it begins to affect her schoolwork or her ability to function. Dr. Katharina Dalton studied a group of English schoolgirls and concluded that premenstrual symptoms resulted in lower grades on examinations; attempts to duplicate her results on several occasions by a researcher at the University of California at Davis, however, were unsuccessful.

The usual response of parents to this type of behavior is to write it off to adolescence; teenagers are difficult. Even when parents do notice a cyclical phenomenon, they don't know what to do about it. Most physicians with whom they raise the issue dismiss it as normal.

Naomi Rath, eighteen, noticed a personality change with her periods when she was sixteen. "I was very moody. Bitchy, I guess you would say. I felt like I was a different person and I didn't like that person very much," she said. "Finally I was having maybe four good days a month." Her mother recalls, "She always had severe, painful periods. She's got every symptom, physical and mental. She'd do and say things she wouldn't ordinarily. She was irritable and angry. She basically is very easy to get along with; she kept it under wraps for a long time. And in between, she would be her own fantastic self. But finally, it was ruining her life. She lost a job over it. This extreme exhaustion would come over her and she couldn't work. And you know, those around you, who deal with you, suffer just as much." After being diagnosed and treated for PMS, Naomi says, "I felt like one hundred pounds had been taken off my shoulders." She was especially glad of the opportunity to meet other women at the center who also had PMS. "It helped a lot in the beginning to talk to the other women," despite the fact that most of them were ten or twenty years older than she. Friends her own age, she says, hadn't been supportive. "When you talk to your girl friends, they laugh and say, 'let's lock YOU up.'"

Her mother says of her daughter, "She doesn't *have* moods anymore. It's a dramatic change. Absolutely."

As the Raths can attest, if the symptoms are severe and last several days, they disrupt relationships with parents, peers, brothers and sisters, teachers. Whether they respond with empathy, anger, or authoritarian control, the girl may begin to act out further, in open rebellion, conflicts with the law, shoplifting, or sometimes by running away or engaging in sex. Some girls, though, become solemn, secretive, and withdraw, not only from their family but also from their friends. This is particularly destructive to self-image at a critical developmental stage.

It's a classic profile, epitomized by the characterization of Frankie Addams, the protagonist of Carson McCullers' *The Member of the Wedding*, a fifteen-year-old girl struggling to deal with her approaching womanhood: "And finally the troubles started. She did things and she

ot herself in trouble. She broke the law. And having once become a
criminal, she broke the law again, and then again. She took the pistol
from her father's bureau drawer and carried it all over town and shot up
the cartridges in a vacant lot. She changed into a robber and stole a
three-way knife from the Sears and Roebuck Store. One Saturday
afternoon she committed a secret and unknown sin. In the MacKeans'
garage, with Barney MacKean, they committed a queer sin, and how
bad it was she did not know. The sin made a shriveling sickness in her
stomach, and she dreaded the eyes of everyone. She hated Barney and
wanted to kill him. Sometimes alone in the bed at night she planned to
shoot him with the pistol or throw a knife between his eyes.''

cting Out

Many adolescents may fantasize, dream, or act out petty rebellions
but take their distress no further. Other adolescents with PMS may
exhibit violent behavior, suicide attempts, alcohol and drug abuse. One
of our patients — let's call her Mara — is a heroin addict. Her parents
noticed monthly episodes of irritability and rebelliousness in her at
puberty, in contrast to her normally happy and outgoing nature. Over
time she withdrew from her friends and was difficult to deal with at
home and at school. The mother kept a diary about her daughter,
documenting the occurrence of these events about every thirty to thirty-
six days. When Mara began to menstruate her periods occurred every
thirty-two to thirty-five days; for several days prior to her period she was
extremely difficult and irritable. At the age of sixteen she became
involved with various types of drugs, rapidly moved on to heroin and
became a heroin addict until we saw her at the age of twenty-six.

Mara told us that she became addicted to heroin for many reasons, but
an important factor was that it was the only substance that satisfactorily
controlled her severe premenstrual symptoms, including depression and
irritability, breast swelling and tenderness, fluid retention with abdominal bloating. When she began to menstruate, she struggled to cope with
these symptoms two weeks out of each month. After trying to block out
the pain with a variety of drugs, including alcohol, she eventually found
that heroin worked. Her addiction landed her in jail on several occasions, for drunk driving and driving while under the influence of drugs;
many times she berated or attempted to challenge the police, which

resulted in additional charges of resisting arrest. Both mother and daughter noted that within a few days of her arrests, the mother would have to bring Tampax to the jail for her daughter.

Mara said the only time she did not crave heroin was during her two pregnancies; she felt "the best I've ever felt," in the second and third trimesters, when enormous amounts of progesterone were floating in her bloodstream, inducing a surge of beta-endorphins that mimicked the heroin high.

PMS can be a nagging source of conflict between a girl and her parents, but particularly between a girl and her mother. The erratic, but cyclical behavior patterns create a bewildering situation, ripe for hostility and misinterpretation. A girl with PMS also may have a tremendously heightened sex drive in the premenstrual phase and may act out sexually or appear to compete with the mother on a sexual level. This is true whether or not the mother has PMS or whether the mother has realized that the daughter's problem rears its head on a monthly basis. If the mother also has the symptoms of PMS, the daughter's behavior compounds her problems and strains the relationship between them. A family with an adolescent suffering from PMS may need psychotherapy or counseling to help them resolve their problems.

Chapter 18

"The time which we have at our disposal every day is elastic; the passions that we feel expand it, those that we inspire contract it; and habit fills up what remains."

Marcel Proust, **Remembrance of Things Past**

The Twenties and Thirties

Time is what there's never enough of in our busy lives, but its constraints may be most bridling to those in their twenties and thirties.

The twenties is a decade of experimentation and experience, the period in which we emerge from our school years and ties to parents, ready to test our wings and shoot for the moon. But it's also a comforting stretch of time in which we are still allowed to make mistakes — in our personal lives or in our occupations — without placing our entire future in jeopardy. The twenties, in fact, is a luxurious span that can spell playtime for those of us who have trouble facing adulthood. And for the ambitious, it's a fertile period for out-achieving colleagues and slipping onto the fast track.

For women committed to a fast-track career course, this is a time of immersion in work and learning from mentors. While the work can be demanding and difficult, neophytes usually don't have to bear the brunt of responsibility for major projects or deals because they're still in training. Thus, there's some freedom and probably time to frolic on occasion.

For women who marry early or are settled into a solid relationship, this the early nesting time — a lot like playing house for some.

For those who choose to start families immediately, this may be a harried but enjoyable time as they grow into their new roles and adapt to the presence of children in their lives.

The clock is no longer a friend as we wind up our twenty-ninth year. Just a turn of the calendar page away is the thirties — the "deadline decade," as Gail Sheehy tells us in *Passages,* a time to climb the job ladder, settle down, raise a family, write that novel, star in a movie, seize center stage of Carnegie Hall or center field of Yankee Stadium, indulge whims and fantasies, accomplish all the dreams we've treasured from childhood — before it's too late, before we tumble headlong into an abyss marked "middle age " as helplessly as Alice cascaded through the rabbit hole. The greatest pressures and highest expectations emerge in our thirties, radiating from all sources — self, mate, children, employer, friends, and community.

For women focusing singlemindedly on a career, the thirties are the critical years for advancement.

For women in a marriage or serious relationship, it's a period requiring substantial attention to their mate.

For women who have young children, this is a nurturing phase when hours must be devoted to the hugging, loving, story-telling, teaching, feeding, washing, tending chores of little ones.

Superwoman's Dilemma

For the superwomen, doing it all simultaneously, the competing demands seem never to stop: mate, children, household, job. Oh, yes, and self. Finding time to read a book or soak in a hot tub is either impossible or the minutes are stolen away from essentials, like doing the laundry or answering a week's worth of mail.

The clock ticks on, a monotonous pressure building up second by second like steam rising in a cast-iron boiler on an icy morning. We become fixated by time as surely as the White Rabbit worried over his pocket watch. The experience is not unique to modern society. Thomas Hardy sounded the theme in *Jude the Obscure:* "As you got older, and felt yourself to be at the center of your time, and not at a point in its circumference as you felt when you were little, you were seized with a sort of shuddering."

What if we can't accomplish it all? What if we face the bathroom mirror one day and look into the eyes of a thirty-five-year-old unhappy in love, unhappy in work, unhappy in the rat race, burnt-out, anxious, and insecure? Even Ralph Waldo Emerson knew that feeling, noting in his *Journals* that "after thirty, a man wakes up sad every morning, excepting perhaps five or six, until the day of his death." The pressures are undeniably real. But most are unrealistic or unnecessary. What begins to happen in the thirties is that the successful adapters approach the pressures in their lives like a cardplayer dealing a game of solitaire: match up the sequences that lead to a winning run and discard the ones that don't. We have to distinguish the pressures that are important and deserve a response from the ones that are unnecessary baggage. The latter are best jettisoned immediately if we're to reach our destination. For many, even the destination has been changed. When we hit the thirties, if we haven't made it past the audition, we have to reassess our goals. The goal should be a happy and fulfilling life. That's not a brass ring restricted to the best and the brightest. We can all find some joy and enjoyment if we're willing to accept our lives. Be good at what you do and be happy with your friends and family. Accept life for what it is, stop demanding the impossible. More importantly, let others know they can't demand the impossible from you.

For women who bear the added burden of premenstrual syndrome, the pressures mount and multiply tenfold because they are dealing with a chronic illness as well as dozens of conflicting demands. Few women in their twenties have severe cases of PMS — they probably haven't encountered as many of the incidents that magnify the risk and intensity of the disorder as women ten or fifteen years older. Many women in this age group who develop PMS may have mild or moderate conditions that can be alleviated by a change in diet, exercise, reduction of stress, and so on.

Highest Risk Group

Women in their thirties constitute the highest risk group for premenstrual syndrome simply because they have probably encountered more of the incidents that are known to contribute to PMS: they are more likely to have been on the birth control pill at some point, to have been pregnant or miscarried, to have had an abortion or tubal ligation or hysterectomy. Those that actually have PMS must decide how to deal with the pressures of job, home, and family. Pressure creates stress, and stress makes any illness worse because it strains the body's flight or fight response and immune system. Those with mild and moderate cases of PMS, which appear one to four days a month, may find that they can fulfill their commitments and juggle all demands merely by making lifestyle changes in diet and exercise and by learning how to relax. They might be able to schedule difficult duties or delicate projects into their symptom-free days. But women with severe PMS have a much more difficult time coping. For them, PMS is a chronic, almost crippling condition that affects one to three weeks of their life each month.

The career woman who is strongly affected by premenstrual syndrome is usually in her late twenties or early thirties. That is a crucial time for job development, the period in which one can make or break a reputation and win promotions. A working woman, whether married or single, is less willing to put up with the symptoms than a woman who doesn't work because she cannot afford to lose time to an illness. The careerist usually is much quicker to seek therapy; she usually searches out treatment before she reaches forty.

Women who are married, whether or not they work outside the home, have added pressures as well as added support systems because of the relationship. By the time a woman is in her thirties she may have been married for five or more years. That's a critical period in which many marriages run into problems requiring time and attention. Women without children are usually involved in a career and face the double load of marital and job pressures. Those who are mothers without jobs probably have young children, who have enormous needs for parental attention and love. The woman with one or two children who develops PMS after pregnancy is in for an especially difficult time. She'll become less joyous around the infant in the face of PMS and the difficulties she faces in meeting all of her responsibilities. Everyone depends on her and she feels that she can't let them down. The wife and mother who doesn't work outside the home, however, can sometimes tolerate PMS longer because she has more supports. She may not seek treatment as aggressively as a woman who works because, unconstrained by office deadlines, she recovers from her symptom days, and like a whirlwind accomplishes everything she left undone as well as the future jobs. Husband and children, even other relatives and friends, may pitch in and help out when she's ill or bedridden. She may develop a convenient amnesia that lets her forget during her good days how painful the symptom days were. As a result, it may take months or years to face up to the fact of recurring illness. The woman who is a wife and mother and maintains a job outside the home has to have a highly refined coping mechanism to manage it all. And many women do; many of them are our patients.

The range of reactions women have to their symptoms is as broad as their personality types. Those who have strong, supportive relationships and seek treatment tend to be able to follow the lifestyle changes and progesterone therapy plans and recover with alacrity. Those without a good support system and with lots of stress in their daily routine — due to marital problems, divorce, separation, or the single life — usually have a lowered tolerance for stress that interferes with their concentration, willpower and discipline. This makes it difficult or impossible for them to follow the diet and other lifestyle changes. Women with PMS need support and help as they approach their treatment: the love and understanding of mate and family, a compassionate and caring personal physician, the motivation and opportunity of a job, profession or school to further their development in this phase of life.

Chapter 19

> *"Life begins at forty."*
>
> Adage

> *"Forty is deep old age. It's indecent,*
> *vulgar, and immoral to live beyond forty."*
>
> Dostoevsky, Notes From the Underground

The Forties

The middle passage of a journey may turn out to be as comfortingly calm as a cup of cocoa sipped by a fire, or mined with as many hazards as the desert sands of El Alamein. The middle years of life's trek bear the same double-edge. A certain confidence acquired along with the bruises of arduous travel is worn by women in their forties, at last settled into careers and personal relationships. After a few digressions of lifestyle, jobs, or mates, they finally know where they're headed. As Jung wrote of life's midpoint, "... we have achieved a real independence and with it, to be sure, a certain isolation. In a sense we are alone, for our 'inner freedom' means that a love relation can no longer fetter us; the other sex has lost its magic power over us, for we have come to know its essential traits in the depths of our own psyche. We shall not easily 'fall in love,' for we can no longer lose ourselves in someone else, but we shall be capable of a deeper love, a conscious devotion to the other." He concludes: "To be sure, it takes half a lifetime to arrive at this stage." Many women can vouch for the fact that it wasn't easy to get here. But having made their peace with the past, they fashion vital, albeit very different, lives.

Beth Davis, forty-six, and her husband, Dennis, the parents of six, have lived with PMS since their marriage began twenty-seven years ago. Davis was referred for treatment to us almost two years ago by a gynecologist who had read about premenstrual syndrome and thought her condition fit the criteria. Since she began responding to the progesterone and lifestyle program, Davis has started a small boutique in her

175

community and joined in a range of social activities that she hadn't bee
well enough to enjoy in her twenties and thirties. "There's so much t
do now, and I'm going to do it all. Dennis and I are having a wonderfu
time together, sharing our fun times and sharing our work. And ou
youngest daughter is having a much easier, less tense childhood than he
older brothers and sisters had. Life does begin at forty — well, in m
case, it was forty-four."

Approaching Menopause

The forties are an emotionally-loaded decade for many wome
because the decade marks the approach to menopause, the end of thei
reproductive years. The *angst* many women express over reaching th
forties is not simply regret or dismay over the loss of youth but a virule
passion stemming from what some perceive to be an outrage unjustl
handed down from Olympus, the threatened theft of their sexuality. Th
sensitivity of women to age is a cliche that has fed a thousand quips ov
the years. Perhaps the best of the worst is that of Ambrose Bierce wh
observed: "You are not permitted to kill a woman who has wronge
you, but nothing forbids you to reflect that she is growing older even
minute. You are avenged 1440 times a day." Cliches are born of reality
like it or not. That's really what the sensitivity of women to age is a
about. It's not the years themselves that count so much, it's th
significance of the aging process for women. Men remain capable c
siring children until they are senile; women are deprived of thei
generative powers at an early age because nature deemed that thei
bodies wouldn't be able to support a fetus to term in the later year
Some women still fear the approach of the forties: as if a woman who i
sensual and desirable woman at thirty-nine is somehow transformed
year or two or three or five later into a dried-up crone. The fears are r
diculous, but their presence cannot be ignored. Women in their fift
decade have developed strengths of emotion, mind, and character tha
enhance their desirability, rather than detract from it. For women wi
premenstrual syndrome, the forties is a time in which the extremes c
their symptoms may lessen naturally, for physiological and soci
reasons. Women of this age may find the pressures on them from fami
and job easing: their children are probably older, in their teens c
twenties, requiring less minute-to-minute supervision and making few

er demands for attention. These women are likely to be further along in their careers than a woman in her thirties, or alternatively, to be resuming a career now that the children are more independent. In either instance, they are unlikely to be precisely at that make-or-break stage, scrambling for promotions and projects as validation of their worth. Children and jobs are two great pressures on women in their thirties that make PMS intolerable. These two stresses are usually absent or minor in the lives of women in their forties. Even the anathema of approaching menopause has proved to be a saving grace. Slowly but surely the secretion of estrogen by the ovaries diminishes in the forties, accompanied by a diminishing of the symptoms associated with estrogen: abdominal bloating, headaches, migraine, epilepsy, fluid retention, and cyclic emotional disturbances.

For most women with premenstrual syndrome, even untreated, the forties is usually the beginning of the end. The worst is over in terms of severity and duration of symptoms, and for most women PMS will end with menopause.

Chapter 20

*"The process of maturing is an art to be
learned, an effort to be sustained. By
the age of fifty you have made yourself
what you are, and if it is good, it is
better than your youth."*

Marya Mannes, More in Anger

Menopause and
Post-Menopause

Reminders of mortality, like dunning notices from creditors, provoke
reactions as predictable as the plot of a Gothic romance: dread, fear,
avoidance, depression, or reluctant confrontation. For women, the start
of menopause signals a harsh reality: fertility is drawing to an end, the
autumn of life is at hand, what Anne Sexton called the "November of
the body." The shock is at least partly absorbed by the length of the
process; menopause spans three to seven years for many women. It's a
shock nonetheless. Doris Lessing's heroine of *The Summer Before the
Dark*, Kate Brown, a middle-aged wife and mother who reclaims her
independence and vitality one summer before her own autumn begins,
considered the situation thus: "Growing old is a matter of years. You
are young, and then you are middle-aged, but it is hard to tell the
moment of passage from one state to the next." She came to this
moment wearily, after some trying and irritating incidents with her
casually philandering husband and four college-age children. When she
reacted to the hostility and aloofness of her children by defiantly
adopting a stray cat and lavishing attention upon it, Lessing writes:
"Just the thing for the menopause,' she had heard Tim say to Eileen.
She had not started the menopause, but it would have been no use saying
so: it had been useful apparently, for the family's mythology, to have a
mother in the menopause."

179

The physical signs start in the forties, a time when some men that age are still dating twenty-year-olds. The menstrual cycles gradually decrease in length. At fifteen, the average cycle is thirty-five days; at twenty-five, it is thirty days; at thirty-five, twenty-eight days. Between forty and fifty, the cycle often shortens to twenty-one days. Then some cycles are missed, some are shorter, some are longer. The extreme irregularity of the cycles is confusing and frustrating to some women; usually the cycles have a clear-cut beginning but an uncertain end. Ovulation may still occur, but with diminishing frequency as estrogen levels ebb to a point where egg follicles are no longer stimulated. Slowly the transition from normal menstruation to permanent amenorrhea is completed: no longer is the month heralded with a flow of blood. Most women with PMS find their symptoms end at or after menopause, but despite the label "premenstrual syndrome," a small percentage of women who reach menopause or are post-menopausal do exhibit the cyclical and recurring symptoms. About ten percent of our patients have been through menopause but exhibit symptoms in a pattern that matches their earlier menstrual cycles. Our oldest patient was fifty-eight when she came to our office for treatment; she had been through menopause five or six years earlier but still had severe PMS. She was successfully treated with progesterone.

Delaying Menopause

Menopause used to occur around age forty, but women now are more likely to experience it at fifty or fifty-one. Women's longer reproductive life, with earlier puberty and menarche and delayed menopause, has evolved with improvements in nutrition and health care. In the 19th Century, menopause struck early. Elizabeth Barrett Browning, then a thirty-nine-year-old spinster, lamented her age and alluded to the rapid approach of menopause in the *Sonnets from the Portuguese,* in phrases like "colors fading," and an analogy to herself, a "casement broken in,/The bats and owlets builders in the roof!" Despite her gloomy outlook she conceived five times during her subsequent marriage to Robert Browning, producing a son amid four miscarriages.

Reproach does not emanate only from the women themselves. Throughout literature, women in the middle years are reviled or worse for their declining fertility. Autumn's approach is again a theme in

William Faulkner's *A Light in August,* where Joanna Burden is anxious over her waning reproductive years. When she thinks she is pregnant she happily tells her lover, Joe Christmas. But when it turns out to have been a false alarm, he strikes her, saying: "There is not anything the matter with you except being old. You just got old and it (menopause) happened to you and now you are not any good any more."

The obsession with fertility and making babies is primeval; two Biblical "miracles" are the reversals of the barrenness of Sarah, the wife of Abraham, and Elizabeth, the cousin of Mary and wife of Zacharias.

The depression, irritability, lowered self-esteem, crying spells, and flaring tempers that frequently accompany the onset of menopause have long been thought to be due to psychological factors — the primordial concern about fertility and the natural reaction to its end — rather than to endocrine changes. Women with PMS, though, may exhibit these symptoms cyclically because of their illness. Estrogen therapy may alleviate some of the psychological problems associated with menopause, but may exacerbate the symptoms of premenstrual syndrome.

Menopause is the grand finale of a gradual process of reproductive burn-out. By the age of fifty, most women have become too old to reproduce and sustain life. The body's store of follicles — which numbered two million at birth and about three hundred thousand at puberty — has simply been depleted. (Most of the follicles die; only about five hundred ever mature into eggs.) The irregular bleeding is the result of stimulation of the remaining follicles, which in turn secrete estrogen. As estrogen levels drop, the remaining follicles increasingly fail to muster the strength to reach ovulation. Without ovulation there's no corpus luteum, no secretion of estrogen and progesterone, no noticeable growth of the endometrium, and no bleeding. The decrease in estrogen takes a toll on the organs that had been nurtured by that hormone. The female reproductive organs wither. Without estrogen the vagina may begin to atrophy and excrete a brownish discharge as its capillaries break down and rupture. The secretion of mucus also dwindles. The uterus begins to shrink because the endometrium is no longer being stimulated by the follicles.

The immediate physiological signs of menopause are hot flashes, which are somehow linked to the loss of estrogen; hot flashes are alleviated by estrogen therapy. The flashes may last only a second or as long as ten minutes; they can be frequent, unsettling, manifested by a sudden sensation of heat or burning, followed by intense perspiration. Usually the flash begins with the sensation of a mild headache or cranial pressure. This quickly mounts to a burning, hot spell that spreads through the upper body with a resulting red flush. Often the flash will permeate the entire body in short, quick waves and the woman's temperature will rise for a moment until the sweating appears, restoring the temperature to normal. Hot flashes may also trigger fatigue, weakness, and dizziness. The mechanism causing the flashes is still unknown.

Estrogen Deficiency and Impact

The most serious health hazard of menopause is osteoporosis, a skeletal disorder where the bones begin to lose mass and strength, becoming brittle and easily broken. This is why the body shrinks with age. Osteoporosis is more common in women than in men; ovarian malfunction is one factor, but the cause of this degenerative disorder remains unknown. Everyone loses bone strength with age, partly due to loss of calcium. But an estrogen deficiency compounds the problem. Short-term estrogen therapy seems to halt the process of bone degeneration and calcium loss. Osteoporosis is a major reason that estrogen therapy is used in postmenopausal women. The risk of heart attacks also increases in women after they reach menopause apparently because estrogen is no longer secreted by the ovaries. But estrogen therapy also carries hazards. One is the increased risk of development of endometrial cancer; another is the elevation of blood pressure which can lead to hypertension. The side effects of estrogen are intolerable for some women: increased vaginal bleeding, breast swelling and tenderness, fluid retention, abdominal bleeding, migraine headaches. Decreasing the estrogen dosage or switching to an estrogen-progestogen program usually eliminates the side effects.

Normal menopausal symptoms — hot flashes, osteoporosis, vaginitis, and the like — are not cyclical. This is how menopausal symptoms can be distinguish from PMS. Some women suffer worse PMS symptoms in the pre-menopause years. We have also seen a few women whose PMS begins at menopause. It usually becomes clear that they had mild PMS prior to menopause, became worse with menopause and worsened afterward. But some really do suffer the onset at menopause. The symptoms tend to be irritability, vague muscle and joint aches, fatigue, lack of concentration, and sometimes excessive use of alcohol. Some doctors who diagnose PMS at this stage treat the menopause in a cycle of progesterone and estrogen (not just one or the other) and think this is the most effective treatment.

The PMS Prescription

Chapter 21

Do You Have PMS?

Premenstrual syndrome is a clinical diagnosis based upon a patient's history; there is no laboratory test that can be done to identify it conclusively. Critics often cite this lack of a biological marker for PMS in their attempts to discredit or downplay it. But these critics, many of them physicians, conveniently ignore the fact that a multitude of "recognized" medical and psychiatric disorders, including depression, are diagnosed from characteristic physical signs, symptoms, and history rather than from lab tests or x-rays. Eventually, with diligent and systematic research, a biological marker may be identified with PMS. So far, though, no research group has taken this issue seriously.

As we have previously explained, the predominance of women experience premenstrual syndrome to some degree. But not all women have it. And most women have only mild cases that do not require medical treatment. Ninety percent of all women who visit our office meet the criteria for a diagnosis of premenstrual syndrome. This is hardly surprising since the women who seek us out are self-selected. Most of them have extensive medical problems of many years' duration, and have been examined and treated by other physicians for their complaints. Only a handful have been accurately diagnosed as having premenstrual syndrome. Many are referred by physicians, either because they are unsure of the diagnosis or have diagnosed it but do not know how to adequately treat PMS. On occasion employers send their employees to us for screening. In the past two years, we have evaluated more than two thousand women from fifty states and half a dozen foreign countries.

About thirty percent of our patients have disorders in addition to PMS, including significant depression, that either have gone undiagnosed or have been misdiagnosed. That's why we carry out a complete physical examination and battery of laboratory and psychological tests on each patient. Some physicians think that these tests aren't necessary. But we think they're extremely telling. Our patients have severe symptoms. Their lives have been disrupted. Virtually all of them have been evaluated previously by other physicians, most by several physicians and several specialists; they usually have had several medications prescribed for them, which have proved ineffective. It is a group that is at high risk for other disorders. We have a responsibility to be cautious, to identify other disorders that may be mimicking PMS, or that should be treated in conjunction with the PMS. One of the caveats of the medical profession is "First, do no harm." This means the physician owes the patient an accurate diagnosis. Our evaluation is tailored to a precise evaluation, physically as well as emotionally. We try to make certain that the patient is treated, or referred for treatment, for all diagnosed disorders, not just PMS.

The most common secondary conditions we observe in our patients are endocrine disorders related to reproduction, including breast and mammary gland conditions, uterine and ovarian disorders, endometriosis, and pelvic inflammatory disease. We've also discovered cases of diabetes, thyroid disease, including thyroid nodules, and allergies. A number of our patients have extensive histories of allergies that haven't been appropriately evaluated or treated. The predominance of thyroid cases and allergies is unusual for the size of the population we've seen; research must be done to explore the possible connection between PMS and these maladies. Other common conditions accompanying PMS are significant clinical depressions, major affective disorders, and atypical depressions, requiring psychotherapy or medication.

Charting Your Symptoms

If you suspect that you may have premenstrual syndrome, the basic monitoring routine to follow requires tracking your physical, psychological, emotional, and behavioral symptoms daily over a two- to three-month period, and maintaining daily weight and temperature records.

For at least one complete menstrual cycle, we recommend that each morning upon arising you take your temperature with a basal (morning) rectal thermometer. A regular fever thermometer is not as accurate as the basal type and won't be as precise. Basal thermometers can be purchased at most pharmacies. The temperature record can be a useful tool in identifying the various stages of the menstrual cycle and can indicate whether ovulation has occurred. Many women tell us that keeping a temperature chart helps them understand their menstrual cycle and correlate their symptoms to it.

Next, you should empty your bladder and weigh yourself without clothes, recording your weight on the chart provided. This record will show whether you are retaining fluids. Symptoms such as abdominal bloating, breast swelling and tenderness, puffiness of the fingers, hands, ankles or around the eyes, backache, sinusitis, and headaches have been attributed to the retention of fluid. Our findings coincide with those of other researchers who report that only about thirty percent of the women who have these symptoms actually retain fluids. Research studies show that many women with PMS do not retain fluids; rather they undergo a redistribution of fluids already in their body during the premenstrual phase.

The symptom check list that follows should be filled out at approximately the same time each day. The list includes the most common complaints and symptoms of women with PMS. In addition we've included the signs of dysmenorrhea and other unrelated complaints, as part of our total monitoring program.

We ask our patients to have someone who lives with them or sees them every day independently to keep track of their observations of the patient's behavior and symptoms as a kind of double-check for accuracy.

We ask patients visiting our office for the first time to bring along the charts — of temperature, weight, and symptom check lists. By the time our patients arrive at the center, they have been keeping these records for one to six weeks. We will not make a diagnosis of PMS until two months of charts, or two complete menstrual cycles, have been maintained and reviewed by us.

During the first visit, which lasts four to six hours, we take extensive histories: a medical history to discern past illnesses, treatments, surgery, medications, and allergic reactions, a psychosocial history of the key events and stresses of the patient's life and her reactions to them, and a lifestyle history of diet and nutritional patterns, exercise, smoking, alcohol consumption, and drug use.

Then the patient is examined by a physician who reviews all this data, asks further questions, and reviews the body systems. Then a complete physical examination is carried out, including a pelvic examination and

DAILY WEIGHT CHART

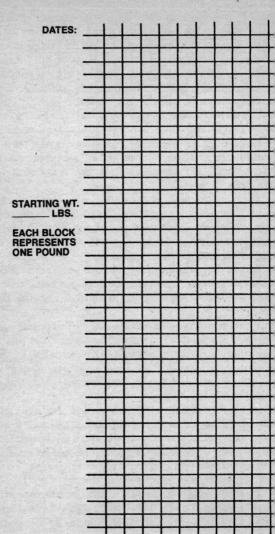

DATES:

STARTING WT.
_____ LBS.

EACH BLOCK
REPRESENTS
ONE POUND

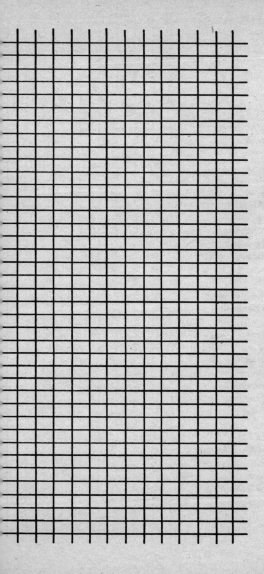

MENSTRUAL CYCLE SYMPTOM SCALE

	Absent	Barely Noticeable	Mild	Moderate	Strong	Severe	Incapacitating
1. Irritability	0	1	2	3	4	5	6
2. Leg Heaviness	0	1	2	3	4	5	6
3. Backache	0	1	2	3	4	5	6
4. Accidents	0	1	2	3	4	5	6
5. Diarrhea	0	1	2	3	4	5	6
6. Fatigue	0	1	2	3	4	5	6
7. Cramps (uterine or pelvic)	0	1	2	3	4	5	6
8. Affectionate	0	1	2	3	4	5	6
9. Abdominal Bloating or Swelling	0	1	2	3	4	5	6
10. Vaginal Discharge, watery	0	1	2	3	4	5	6
11. Vaginal Discharge, thick	0	1	2	3	4	5	6
12. Eye Pain	0	1	2	3	4	5	6
13. Difficulty Concentrating	Y	5	6	7	8	9	0
14. Increased Energy	0	1	2	3	4	5	6
15. Insomnia	0	1	2	3	4	5	6
16. Hives (rashes)	0	1	2	3	4	5	6
17. Clumsiness or Incoordination	0	1	2	3	4	5	6
18. Sore Throat	0	1	2	3	4	5	6
19. Tingling in Hands	0	1	2	3	4	5	6
20. Acne-like Eruptions	0	1	2	3	4	5	6
21. Poor Judgment	0	1	2	3	4	5	6
22. Orderliness	0	1	2	3	4	5	6
23. Panic Attack	0	1	2	3	4	5	6
24. Sharp One-Sided Ovarian Pain	0	1	2	3	4	5	6
25. Asthma Attack	0	1	2	3	4	5	6
26. Cravings for Sweet Foods	0	1	2	3	4	5	6
27. Headaches (Migraine)	0	1	2	3	4	5	6
28. Headaches (Tension)	0	1	2	3	4	5	6
29. Increased Arguments	0	1	2	3	4	5	6

	Absent	Barely Noticeable	Mild	Moderate	Strong	Severe	Incapacitating
30. Nausea and/or Vomiting	0	1	2	3	4	5	6
31. Breast Swelling	0	1	2	3	4	5	6
32. Vaginal Spotting	0	1	2	3	4	5	6
33. Menstrual Flow	0	1	2	3	4	5	6
34. Loneliness	0	1	2	3	4	5	6
35. Muscle Stiffness	0	1	2	3	4	5	6
36. Dull Abdominal Aching	0	1	2	3	4	5	6
37. Decreased Hearing Ability	0	1	2	3	4	5	6
38. Difficulty Using Contact Lens	0	1	2	3	4	5	6
39. Fear of Losing Control	0	1	2	3	4	5	6
40. Sinusitis	0	1	2	3	4	5	6
41. Craving for Salty Foods	0	1	2	3	4	5	6
42. Increased Sex Drive	0	1	2	3	4	5	6
43. Decreased Work/School Performance	0	1	2	3	4	5	6
44. Increased Need to Sleep	0	1	2	3	4	5	6
45. Feelings of Suffocation	0	1	2	3	4	5	6
46. Excitement	0	1	2	3	4	5	6
47. Conjunctivitis (itchy red eye)	0	1	2	3	4	5	6
48. Weight Gain	0	1	2	3	4	5	6
49. Forgetfulness	0	1	2	3	4	5	6
50. Leg Cramps or Tenderness	0	1	2	3	4	5	6
51. Decreased Sex Drive	0	1	2	3	4	5	6
52. Stay Home From Work/School	0	1	2	3	4	5	6
53. Painful or Tender Breasts	0	1	2	3	4	5	6
54. Cold Sweats							
55. Inefficiency	0	1	2	3	4	5	6

	Absent	Barely Noticeable	Mild	Moderate	Strong	Severe	Incapacitating
56. Depression (sad or blue)	0	1	2	3	4	5	6
57. Runny Nose (rhinorrhea)	0	1	2	3	4	5	6
58. Ankle Swelling	0	1	2	3	4	5	6
59. Sores in Mouth	0	1	2	3	4	5	6
60. Decreased Alcohol Tolerance	0	1	2	3	4	5	6
61. Constipation	0	1	2	3	4	5	6
62. Suspiciousness/Paranoid	0	1	2	3	4	5	6
63. Anger	0	1	2	3	4	5	6
64. Crying Spells	0	1	2	3	4	5	6
65. Heart Pounding	0	1	2	3	4	5	6
66. Finger Swelling	0	1	2	3	4	5	6
67. Mood Swings	0	1	2	3	4	5	6
68. Chest Pains	0	1	2	3	4	5	6
69. Hot Flashes	0	1	2	3	4	5	6
70. Numbness and Tingling in Feet	0	1	2	3	4	5	6
71. Confusion	0	1	2	3	4	5	6
72. Burst of Activity	0	1	2	3	4	5	6
73. Distractable	0	1	2	3	4	5	6
74. Increased Alcohol Consumption	0	1	2	3	4	5	6
75. Joint Pains	0	1	2	3	4	5	6
76. Seizures	0	1	2	3	4	5	6
77. Increased Need for Religion	0	1	2	3	4	5	6
78. Anxiety	0	1	2	3	4	5	6
79. Increased Thirst	0	1	2	3	4	5	6
80. Dizziness or Faintness	0	1	2	3	4	5	6
81. Avoid Social Activities	0	1	2	3	4	5	6
82. Restlessness	0	1	2	3	4	5	6
83. Ringing in Ears	0	1	2	3	4	5	6

	Absent	Barely Noticeable	Mild	Moderate	Strong	Severe	Incapacitating
84. General Aches & Pains	0	1	2	3	4	5	6
85. Tenseness	0	1	2	3	4	5	6
86. Vaginal Itching	0	1	2	3	4	5	6
87. Facial Swelling	0	1	2	3	4	5	6
88. Aggressiveness							
89. Hit Someone or Something	0	1	2	3	4	5	6
90. Indecision	0	1	2	3	4	5	6
91. Decreased Appetite	0	1	2	3	4	5	6
92. Blind Spots, Fuzzy Vision	0	1	2	3	4	5	6
93. Bladder Infection	0	1	2	3	4	5	6
94. Sensitivity to Light	0	1	2	3	4	5	6
95. Increased Sensitivity to Noise	0	1	2	3	4	5	6
96. Stye	0	1	2	3	4	5	6
97. Increased Frequency of Urination	0	1	2	3	4	5	6
98. Decreased Frequency of Urination	0	1	2	3	4	5	6
99. Bruising	0	1	2	3	4	5	6
100. Sense of Well Being	0	1	2	3	4	5	6
101. (Other) _____	0	1	2	3	4	5	6

Number of Suppositories Used Today _____

Morning Weight _____

Pap smear. Appropriate laboratory tests are then ordered, including a complete blood count, urinalysis, a chemical profile in which various biochemical factors in the body are screened, a fasting blood-sugar level, and a two-hour postprandial blood-sugar test for diabetes. We also measure thyroid function and production of various hormones, including prolactin, follicle-stimulating hormone, luteinizing hormone, progesterone, and estradiol, the major estrogen. Taking these measurements and considering the day of the patient's cycle and her basal temperature, we can make a fair assessment as to the efficiency of the hypothalamic-pituitary-ovarian axis.

The lab studies are not used to diagnose PMS, but to rule out other disorders.

Later we ask the patient to undergo a battery of psychological tests, including the Minnesota Multi-Phasic Personality Inventory, the Beck Depression Inventory, the Bender-Gestalt, Symptom Check List 90-R, or Cornell Medical Index, and an alcohol-use assessment inventory. A psychologist reviews the findings and prepares a profile of each patient, which adds another dimension to the evaluation. It's also a good screening method to rule out patients who have significant psychological problems, assess depth of depression, and identify organic factors that might affect emotional or mental functioning.

We also hold an informational and question-and-answer session of thirty minutes to an hour discussing the history and impact of PMS, lifestyle changes, alternative treatments, and progesterone therapy.

Family Support

At the initial visit, we bring together groups of six to twelve patients and encourage them to bring a relative or friend with them. Most do. This is important because it provides us with an additional source of information about the patient and confirms or expands what we can find out about the course of their illness and their lifestyle. For the relative, husband, or friend, it's an important means of including them in the evaluation and treatment of a condition that has probably intruded into their lives as well. They also find it reassuring to hear the experiences of other women and their families. Relatives frequently want to make certain that the"real story is told," that the extent of the problems for the woman as well as the family is made clear to us. This session is usually the first time these women have found others who understand exactly what they're talking about. Many friendships are made on the first visit that endure over many months and thousands of miles.

One husband from the Southwest told me that he had known in advance how much our evaluation would cost in terms of airfare, hotel, the clinical evaluation and laboratory studies, but he hadn't anticipated bills for long-distance telephone calls. His wife and many of the women she had met at our office, most of whom lived in different parts of the country, were operating an informal support network via telephone.

Following Up

Our patients are asked to maintain the daily records until they return for a second visit, which is scheduled anywhere from two to ten weeks later to ensure that charts for at least two complete menstrual cycles are completed. We insist on at least two complete cycles of charting before making the diagnosis of PMS. This is required to document any case of PMS; it is a belief that is shared by Dr. Katharina Dalton who has been evaluating and treating women with PMS for thirty years.

Usually the patient and our staff will be in contact with each other during this interval once or twice to assess how the patient is doing and answer questions about PMS or the charts. When the patient returns, she often again brings a relative or friend.

During the second visit, the patient meets briefly with a staff member to review the data she has brought, and to review their experiences during the interval since the first visit. Then she is seen by a physician. The physician integrates all the data, reviewing the history, the physical findings, lab data, psychological tests, chart material and such, discusses this with the patient and relative and then makes a diagnosis. We then recommend various ways that the patient may be treated for PMS, in light of individual needs and desires and the needs and desires of the family. Then a treatment program is mapped out, which may include lifestyle changes, nutritional supplementation, counseling, treatment with progesterone, or a combination of these.

Women with other medical disorders are referred for further specialty consultation or psychotherapy or counseling. Nutritional counseling, either in a group situation or individually, may also be required. Perhaps most importantly, we urge all our patients to join a PMS support group for reassurance and bolstering of their attitude and commitment to overcoming PMS.

For many women, maintaining a simple menstrual calendar is helpful, whether in addition to or instead of the detailed menstrual cycle symptom scale included earlier in this chapter. The menstrual calendar that appears here should be maintained daily for at least three months to determine if the pattern of your symptoms fits the diagnosis of premenstrual syndrome.

On each day of your menstrual flow, mark the letter M in the block corresponding to the date of the month. Each day that you experience mild symptoms, whether physical or psychological, pencil in a small x. On days that the symptoms are serious, pencil in a large X. If your symptoms recur in the same pattern, prior to the onset of menstruation, and followed by a symptom-free week, you may have premenstrual syndrome.

Making an accurate diagnosis of PMS is the first step toward eliminating the symptoms. The next step is the patient's. She must make a serious commitment to follow the course of treatment recommended by her physician. Chronic disorders, including premenstrual syndrome, can only be resolved when patients are committed to following a regular and diligent regimen. The commitment must be complete, but women with PMS must realize that they should approach their treatment program one day at a time. Slow but steady progress is the only way to deal with PMS.

MENSTRUAL CALENDAR

Name _____ Year _____

	Jan.	Feb.	Mar.	Apr.	May	Jun.	Jul.	Aug.	Sep.	Oct.	Nov.	Dec.
1												
2												
3												
4												
5												
6												
7												
8												
9												
10												
11												
12												
13												
14												
15												
16												
17												
18												
19												
20												
21												
22												
23												
24												
25												
26												
27												
28												
29												
30												
31												
otal												

Chapter 22

"Anything that might be cured with diet should not be treated by any other means."

Moses Maimonides

The PMS Diet

"Let thy food be thy medicine," adjured Hippocrates more than 2500 years ago. That admonition is well applied to women with PMS, many of whom are overweight, some of whom face monthly cravings for sweet or salty foods. In the initial visit to our office, some of our patients are a little surprised that we are almost as interested in their eating habits as we are in their depressions and hormonal levels. If one applied "you are what you eat," to a premenstrual syndrome sufferer, the profile would be one of more refined carbohydrates, refined sugars, dairy products and sodium, and less zinc, B vitamins, magnesium, manganese, and iron than a woman without PMS. Many women with premenstrual syndrome have food disorders: binge eating is the most common problem, but we have also identified anorexics and bulimics at the center. Eating disorders, depression, and hormonal imbalances make comfortable bedfellows, as we have pointed out in preceding chapters.

Many of our patients on progesterone therapy find a welcome side effect: progesterone, which is known to have a sedative effect on the brain that may ease the panic or hunger sensations that fuel eating binges, helps them stick to a diet and lose weight effortlessly. As Jane Pownter said, "I'm symptom-free except for an occasional craving one day a week, usually the day before I menstruate. I've stuck pretty much to the diet and I've lost about ten pounds. I was dieting when I went there, because I am a big woman, and I'm continuing to lose weight." Greta Minter adds, "I know that I'm going to have to stick with this treatment. The diet I'm on is going to have to be a lifetime thing."

Hypoglycemia and Sugar

In a nation addicted to processed and fast foods and sugar in any form, it is hardly surprising that twenty million to forty million Americans suffer from a nutritional and endocrine imbalance stemming from overdoses of sugar. Hypoglycemia affects more women than men, especially women between thirty and forty years of age. Women in their thirties also constitute the high risk population for premenstrual syndrome. Many women with PMS have been misdiagnosed as suffering from hypoglycemia. We have also seen some women who suffer from hypoglycemia and do not have PMS. But a number of women with PMS do have altered glucose tolerance levels during the luteal phase of their menstrual cycle. That is why we will discuss hypoglycemia here.

The body takes all sugars introduced into its system and changes them into glucose, or blood sugar. Hypoglycemia — literally, low blood sugar — is a condition of faulty glucose metabolism in which an increased production of insulin drains the body of glucose. Because every cell of the body requires glucose to function, the resulting glucose starvation can play havoc with all systems.

Normally, following a meal, there is an immediate rise in the blood sugar level as carbohydrates, including refined sugar, are rapidly metabolized and absorbed into the bloodstream. This escalating level of glucose triggers the production of insulin, a hormone secreted by the pancreas. Insulin removes much of the glucose and stores it in the liver in the form of glycogen for later use as food for the body. In the hypoglycemic, however, the pancreas runs amok, producing too much insulin, which rapidly drains the blood of its glucose supply. Blood sugar levels plummet rapidly and the body becomes starved for food, despite the fact that it has recently been fed.

Most cells in the body can store some glucose. The brain cannot; it depends on a continual supply from the bloodstream. If the brain becomes starved for glucose, it will grow exhausted and misfunction. A healthy diet provides intermittent supplies of carbohydrates, protein, and fat throughout the day — that's why nutritionists usually recommend that people eat three balanced meals daily. The regulation of the body's glucose is controlled by the hypothalamus and involves hormonal secretions, the nervous system, and dietary intake. When the body's sensors indicate to the hypothalamus that a low blood sugar condition — hypoglycemia — exists, this complex system reacts to increase glucose levels in the blood and reduce the amount of glucose sent to the brain and peripheral cells, including muscles. It is this readjustment of the body's balance of glucose that triggers symptoms of hypoglycemia, including faintness, weakness, tremulousness, blurred vision, hunger, palpitations, fast pulse rate, sweating, tightness in the throat, restlessness, irritability, and even anxiety. If the brain is deprived of glucose for a sufficient length of time, other symptoms may occur, including depression, lassitude, headache, forgetfulness, confusion, lack of coordination, and eventually seizures and coma. The hypoglycemic episode ends when enough glucose is released from the liver or when the individual obtains enough glucose from food.

Hypoglycemia is a relative condition. Some individuals diagnosed as hypoglycemic may have low blood sugar levels that actually fall within the normal range. However, their bodies perceive the level to be abnormal and respond with a bombardment of insulin and epinephrine. This is a common occurrence in women with PMS. During the time of their symptoms, there is a change in glucose tolerance. The change may not be strictly interpreted as a hypoglycemic level when compared with normal glucose blood levels but these women's bodies respond as if they were hypoglycemic. The decline in blood sugar level is relative to what their bodies are used to and will increase insulin production.

Fewer than ten percent of our patients have hypoglycemia as well as PMS. However, some of our patients tell us that if they do not eat something every four to six hours during their symptom phase they develop symptoms very like those experienced during the mildest stage of hypoglycemia. Most of these women do not have hypoglycemia. The blood glucose levels of the vast majority of our patients remain in the normal range even during their symptom phase. It appears, though, that they have a lower individual threshold for glucose during their symptom phase, which signals to their body that a hypoglycemic condition exists. The body's reaction to this signal is what triggers the symptoms of hypoglycemia. These symptoms do not appear if these women eat several small meals throughout the day. And these symptoms do not occur during the non-symptom phase of these women's menstrual cycle, even when they fail to eat something every four to six hours.

Hypoglycemia is identified by a glucose tolerance test, which monitors the body's sugar metabolism over several hours, after fasting and after ingesting a large amount of carbohydrates and sugars. Many women with PMS have flattened glucose tolerance curves, indicating an increased tolerance for sugar. Obesity is a frequent complication because the hypoglycemic is often hungry. In recent years, some researchers have suggested a high rate of hypoglycemia among the obese, hyperkinetic children, schizophrenics, alcoholics, drug addicts, and juvenile delinquents.

Stress Worsens Condition

Caffeine, nicotine, and stress exacerbate the hypoglycemic response. Caffeine and nicotine are powerful stimulants that along with stressful situations provoke the generation of adrenalin, which in turn triggers the production of insulin. (One way the body reacts to stress is by lowering blood sugar levels.) As a result, the hypoglycemic may wind up feeling exhausted, hungry, depressed, anxious, and tense. If a lot of refined sugar is then consumed, the effects can be debilitating. The highly refined sugar you eat forces an amino acid into your brain cells where it is converted to serotonin. Too much serotonin may cause nervous tension, palpitation, and drowsiness. Combine stress with a high intake of refined sugar and you set in motion a self-perpetuating cycle.

Refined sugar triggers insulin release but in excess of what is needed. Refined sugar also increases the ability of insulin to act by three to eleven times. In the week before your period, your body is more responsive to insulin. All these factors tend to lower your blood sugar. In some women, the effect of sugar in the diet can be devastating. One of our patients says her preschool-aged children act as her anti-sugar sentries. "They know I can't eat sugar. I have fainted, become very, very irritable and weepy from eating sugar," she explained. "If my daughter sees me going to eat anything with sugar in it, she says 'that's a no-no.' "

Once hypoglycemia is detected, it can be treated with a proper diet. The aim of the diet is to stabilize the blood sugar level, which is why the hypoglycemic should eat several small meals or snacks several times a day rather than one or two or three large meals. Sugar is absorbed into the bloodstream the fastest of all foods. Complex carbohydrates, especially whole grains, nuts, and vegetables, are also converted to glucose after ingestion, but at a slower rate. Proteins and fats are metabolized more slowly as well; consequently the blood sugar rises much more slowly and consistently. The classic hypoglycemic diet substitutes proteins and fats for most of the sugar in a diet.

Some women with the premenstrual syndrome may also be hypoglycemic. But the classic hypoglycemic diet is not ideal for them because it usually contains too much calcium, too many fats, too much protein, and other substances that can exacerbate the symptoms of PMS. To correct the nutritional imbalances most of our patients suffer, we have developed a dietary program that restricts the amount of sugar, sodium, caffeine, dairy products, and red meat, and increases the intake of complex carbohydrates and foods high in the minerals and vitamins women with PMS need.

Our Diet Program

We recommend that women eat six times a day: three meals a day with a mid-morning snack, a mid-afternoon snack, and a snack before bedtime. This isn't a green light for gluttony, however. Women who are at their ideal weight should take in the same number of total calories as they would in three meals. Women who want to lose weight should cut their total daily caloric intake but divide it over six small meals or three meals and three snacks. We suggest that active women who do not need to lose weight restrict their daily intake to 1,500 calories and women who need to lose weight limit themselves to 1,000 calories a day. Consult your physician and/or nutritionist about the appropriateness of the program for your needs.

We recommend that women change their diet to:

1. Restrict themselves to less than three ounces of red meat a day, and limit total protein intake to four ounces of protein on a 1,000-calorie diet or seven ounces of protein on a 1,500-calorie diet. Protein should represent no more than 20 percent of total daily calories. The best sources of protein are fish, poultry, whole grains and legumes. Dairy products — eggs, cheese, milk, yogurt, butter — should be limited to two servings a day.

2. Increase intake of complex carbohydrates to account for 50 to 65 percent of total daily calories, the higher the better.

3. Reduce refined sugar intake to five teaspoonfuls a day. Eliminate candy, chocolate, cake, pie, pastries, and ice cream from your diet. If you must have something sweet, eat fresh fruit.

4. Limit intake of fats to polyunsaturated vegetable oil fats. These should account for less than 20 percent of calories a day.

5. Reduce salt intake to less than three grams a day. Soft drinks, club soda, and tonics — even diet sodas — have large amounts of salt in the form of sodium benzoate. Try drinking seltzer, mineral water, or plain tap water on ice instead.

6. Sharply reduce or eliminate caffeine (coffee, tea, cola drinks, chocolate). Use decaffeinated coffee or tea.

7. Sharply increase the intake of green, leafy vegetables, whole grains, cereals, and legumes.

8. Limit alcohol intake to one ounce of hard liquor a day, four ounces of wine or twelve ounces of beer.

9. Increase the intake of cis-linoleic acid which is contained in safflower oil and other foods. It is a precursor to prostaglandin E-1, which is thought to play a role in some of the symptoms of PMS.

10. Avoid most processed and fast foods, which contain large amounts of salt and sugar and chemicals.

Caffeine

We recommend that a woman reduce the amount of caffeine in her diet because it may increase the body's need for B vitamins. Caffeine is found in coffee, tea, most colas and soda drinks, and in chocolate. Caffeine makes breast symptoms worse — breast swelling, engorgement, and tenderness. It may increase irritability, hyperactivity, and headaches. Many women find that if they reduce or eliminate caffeine that one or another of their symptoms will improve, some to a very significant degree. Even those whose symptoms do not go away find some improvement.

Salt

Women who experience fluid retention — swelling of the face, hands, feet, breasts, weight gain in the days preceding their periods — as part of their premenstrual symptoms should try to eliminate salt from their diet, especially prior to menstruation.

Studies of women suffering from fluid retention have shown that they have elevated levels of hormones of the adrenal glands which control water and salt retention by the kidney. These salt-retaining hormones stimulated when stress and high brain serotonin trigger the release of brain hormone called ACTH. Excess refined carbohydrates increase brain serotonin. And insulin also plays a role. Excess refined carbohydrates trigger insulin release in excess. Insulin is known to prevent the kidneys from excreting salt. Salt and water retention is in part an insulin effect. For many women with PMS, the craving for sweets and subsequent ingestion of large amounts of refined carbohydrates or sugar precede the swelling and weight gain, which seems to confirm the roles of refined sugar-triggered insulin release. Poor nutrition decreases resistance to stress. Stress by itself causes the adrenal glands to release increased amounts of salt-retaining hormones into the blood, adding to the salt-retaining effect of insulin.

Foods To Avoid or Limit — High in Sodium

Processed and fast foods
Potato chips
Pretzels
Corn, taco and tortilla chips

Prepared, preserved or dried, smoked and canned meats and sausages

Frankfurters	Bacon	Ham
Sausage	Kidneys	Brains
Sweetbreads	Corned beef	Pastrami
Pâté	Cold cuts	Herring
Anchovies	Sardines	Lox, or smoked salmon
Sturgeon	Caviar	

Preserved or pickled fish
Canned fish, except that packed in water and low in salt

Artichokes	Beets	Chard
Kale	Frozen peas	Sauerkraut
Frozen lima beans	White turnips	

Condiments:

Mustard	Catsup	Relish
Mayonnaise	Horseradish	Duck sauce
Barbecue sauces	Soy sauce	Pickles
Sweet and sour sauces		Olives
Worcestershire sauce		

Miscellaneous:

Bouillion cubes	Onion salt	Garlic salt
Molasses	Tomato juice	Celery salt and flakes
Instant cocoa	V-8 juice	Meat tenderizers

Magnesium and Calcium

Americans in general, but American women in particular, may have deficiency of magnesium in their diet. Studies by Drs. Guy E. Abraha and Michael M. Lubran in Los Angeles of women with PMS indica that they have even lower magnesium levels than women without PM This could explain some of the common symptoms of PMS such mood swings, nervous tension, bloating and breast tenderness. R searchers have not yet discovered whether PMS causes this deficien or if the deficiency causes PMS symptoms. In any event, an increase magnesium in the diet may reduce PMS symptoms in some wome Magnesium helps calcium absorption and deposition in the bones whe it belongs. But calcium interferes with magnesium absorption. Magn sium decreases the demand for calcium and calcium increases th demand for magnesium. It makes sense, then, to limit the amount calcium in your diet — dairy products — because it interferes wi magnesium absorption. Dairy products have ten times more calciu than magnesium. You should favor foods that have at least as mu magnesium as calcium, with a daily allowance of 300 to 600 milligrar of magnesium.

Many women crave chocolate, which may be a sign of magnesiu deficiency. Chocolate is relatively rich in magnesium and in phenylet ylamine, a substance produced by the brain that is a cousin of amphe amine. Chocolate also contains caffeine, although in much low amounts than coffee or tea. An ounce of bittersweet chocolate contai 5 to 10 milligrams of caffeine, compared with 100 to 150 milligrams caffeine in a cup of brewed coffee.

There are much better sources of magnesium than chocolate: whc grains, green leafy vegetables, legumes, nuts, seeds, cereals, ai shellfish.

We've provided the following list to help you make your choices whole grains and vegetables from those with higher magnesium/ca cium ratios. That doesn't mean that all foods with relatively lc magnesium/calcium ratios are bad — lettuce, for example, has a ratio 0.26 but it's a healthy, vitamin-filled, low-calorie food that is good include in your daily menus.

Magnesium and Calcium Concentrations

	Magnesium (mg/100cal)	Calcium (mg/100cal)	Magnesium/Calcium Ratio
Spinach	315	365	0.86
Cabbage	76	200	0.38
Carrots	55	82	0.67
Tomato	64	61	1.0
Lettuce	63	238	0.26
Potato	45	9	5.0
Lentils	24	24	1.0
Cashew	48	7	7.0
Almond	45	39	1.2
Brazil nut	38	28	1.4
Hazel nut	36	33	1.1
Peanut	30	12	2.4
Chestnut	21	14	1.5
Walnut	20	15	1.34
Pecan	19	11	1.8
Sunflower seed	7	21	0.3
Rye	34	11½	3.0
Wheat	34	11	3.1
Oat	38	18	2.1
Corn	42	6	7.0
Brown rice	25	9	2.8
Barley	11	4.6	2.3
Millet	50	6.2	8.2
Buckwheat	69	34	2.0

Potassium

Potassium is a mineral critical to muscular contraction and nerve stimulation; it also regulates the body's water balance. Inadequate potassium may lead to muscle cramping. The body's concentration of potassium is regulated by the kidneys and requires a proper balance with sodium — salt. Muscle and nerve functioning suffer when there's an imbalance between sodium and potassium. An excess of one will cause the loss of the other in the urine. Diets high in salt lead to potassium deficiency. Women who take diuretics to prevent fluid retention, bloating, and weight gain before their periods may well be depleting their potassium reserves. Individuals with high blood pressure, diabetes, or liver disease also are high risks for potassium deficiency.

Bananas, oranges, orange juice, broccoli, lettuce, melons, wheat germ, unsalted peanuts, lentils, dates, potatoes, and squash are good sources of potassium. Hypoglycemia may result in a loss of potassium. It is important to add these foods to your diet. The recommended daily allowance of potassium is two to five grams.

Zinc

Of all the minerals in the body, zinc is one of the most important. It plays a major role in the synthesis of proteins and DNA and RNA; it is required for cell growth and the formation of connective tissues; it is a factor in forty or more enzyme reactions. Without zinc, for example, the carbon dioxide exchange in the cells could not be accomplished fast enough to keep a human alive. Zinc acts as the traffic cop of the cells and surrounding membranes, policing the metabolism of other minerals, including copper, magnesium, manganese, and selenium.

An excess of copper in the system can lead to zinc deficiency. In the United States, most drinking water passes through copper plumbing pipes, most over-the-counter vitamin supplements contain copper but not zinc, and freshly grown fruits and vegetables are harvested from soil severely deficient in zinc. Zinc deficiency is a common condition in women, especially those with copper IUDs. Some researchers report that the level of copper is high and that of zinc is low one week before the menstrual period when women are more liable to depressive disorders. Zinc levels can also be disturbed by estrogen, which is why women taking oral contraceptives may have zinc-related problems. A 1972 study found that estrogen raises the level of copper in the bloodstream and lowers that of zinc. Also, diuretics deplete zinc levels. If you take water pills for salt retention you may require zinc supplements.

The best sources of zinc are liver, mushrooms, milk, eggs, red meat, brewer's yeast, nuts, legumes, and seafood, especially oysters and herring. The recommended daily requirement is 15 milligrams for adults, 20 milligrams for pregnant women, and 25 milligrams for lactating women.

To help you plan your daily menus we've included the following calorie/portion guidelines.

Remember, if you're trying to lose weight, try to limit your daily caloric intake to 1,000 calories. If you want to maintain your weight, use 1,500 calories as your limit.

Protein

On a 1,500 calorie diet, you can include seven ounces of protein and a maximum of two dairy servings a day, with only three ounces of the protein represented by red meat. On a 1,000 calorie diet, you can include four ounces of protein, of which red meat can constitute only three ounces; again limit your dairy products servings to two.

Meat and meat substitutes contain 55 calories per ounce, seven grams of protein per ounce, three grams of fat per ounce.

The meat substitutes we are including are 1 egg, not fried; ¼ cup of Fleishman's Egg Beaters (low-cholesterol egg substitute), and ½ cup uniform cottage cheese.

> 1 oz. low sodium cheese is equal to 1 oz. of meat and 1 serving of fat.
> ½ cup creamed cottage cheese is equal to 2 oz. of meat and 1 serving of fat.
> 2 tbsp. peanut butter without salt is equal to 1 oz meat and 2 servings of fat.
> If the meat you choose is marbled in fat, omit 1 serving of fat for each 1 oz. meat you eat.
> ¼ cup of canned tuna fish, packed in water and low in sodium equals one ounce of meat.
> ¼ cup of unsalted salmon equals one ounce of meat.
> Try to choose your protein servings from the above or from:

Poultry — chicken, turkey, cornish hen (remove skin)
Veal — especially the leg, loin and shoulder, cutlets (avoid patties; they usually include beef fat)
Fresh white fish (frozen is too salty)
Lamb — steak, leg, chop (trim all fat)
Beef — only lean cuts such as tenderloin, rump, round steak or roast, London broil, braciole, eye of round, 90 percent lean hamburger
Pork — sometimes the loin is lean enough

Dairy products (limit to two servings a day)
> See egg servings above
> 1 serving equals 4 ounces of skim milk,
> or low fat yoghurt without sugar or fruit,

or 2 ounces of evaporated skim milk
or 4 ounces of buttermilk.

Starch
1 serving equals 70 calories, 15 grams of carbohydrate and 2 grams of protein

> One serving equals
> 1 slice white, rye, raisin or wheat bread
> 1 small roll (16 rolls to the pound)
> 1 ounce (saucer size) pita or Syrian bread

The following rolls weigh about 2 oz and are equal to 2 servings of starch and 140 calories:

> Hamburger roll
> Frankfurter roll
> Bagel
> English muffin

The following breads only weigh ½ ounce a slice. Two slices are equal to one serving of starch:

> Hollywood
> Weight Watcher's
> Melba Thin (Arnold or Pepperidge Farm)
> All of the following equal 1 serving of starch:
> 1 tortilla
> 1 matzoh (six-inch round)
> 5 Melba toast rectangles
> 8 Melba toast rounds (half dollar size)
> 25 unsalted pretzel sticks
> 4 Uneeda Biscuits
> 3 Zwieback Toast
> 2 bread sticks (unsalted, 8 inches long)
> 3 cups unsalted popcorn (no added fat)
> 6 salt-free Venus Wafers
> 4 Arrowroot cookies
> 3 Ginger snaps
> 5 Vanilla wafers
> 3 Lorna Doone shortbread cookies
> 1½ inch square of angel or sponge cake
> 2 Graham crackers

½ cup Jello (with sugar)
2 tbsp cornstarch
2 tbsp flour
3 tbsp cornflake crumbs
1½ tbsp uncooked barley
¼ cup Graham cracker crumbs
¾ cup unfrosted cereals
¼ cup wheat germ
½ cup cooked cereal (unsalted)
½ cup dried beans or dried peas (cooked and unsalted)
⅓ cup whole kernel frozen corn (unsalted or canned without salt or sugar)
1 6-inch ear of corn, no salt in the water
½ cup frozen lima beans (unsalted)
⅔ cup fresh parsnips (unsalted)
½ cup frozen peas (unsalted, frozen or canned without salt or sugar)
1 small unsalted potato (about size of tennis ball)
½ cup mashed potato (not instant, unsalted)
¾ cup fresh pumpkin (unsalted)
½ cup fresh or frozen winter squash (unsalted)
½ cup pasta (noodles, spaghetti, macaroni; unsalted)
½ cup rice, cooked (unsalted)

The following foods contain more fat than other starches and more calories (about 115 calories per serving). They equal 1 starch and 1 fatty food per serving.

1 waffle or pancake (about size of saucer)
8 unsalted French fried potatoes
1 small muffin (without salt or sugar)
1 small biscuit (without salt or sugar)

Fatty Foods
Our nutritional program limits fats to about 20 percent or less of total calories.

1 serving contains 5 grams fat and 45 calories. (All nuts and seeds should be salt free):

1 tsp butter
1 tsp margarine

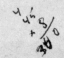

⅛ avocado
1 tsp oil (any; but corn oil and safflower oil are better)
2 tsp Miracle Whip
1 tsp mayonnaise
1 tbsp almonds
2 Brazil nuts
5 Filbert nuts
1 tsp pecans
1½ tbsp pine nuts or pignolis
15 pistachio nuts
1 tbsp walnuts
1 tbsp pumpkin seeds
2 tsp sesame seeds
2 tbsp coffee cream (light)
2 tbsp sour cream
1 tbsp heavy cream (whipping cream)
1 tbsp cream cheese

Our nutritional program requires patients to make complex carbohydrates account for 50 to 65 percent of total calories — the higher the better. The following fruits and vegetables are complex carbohydrates.

Vegetables
One serving equals one-half cup of fresh or frozen vegetables, no salt added. Dietetic canned or no salt vegetables may also be used. Avoid sauerkraut. Do not add salt in cooking.

Asparagus	Greens (chard, kale, spinach, collards, mustard, beet, dandelion)	
Bean sprouts	Lettuce (all kinds, no limit on servings)	
Beets	Mushrooms	
Broccoli	Okra	
Brussel sprouts	Rhubarb	
Cabbage	Rutabaga	Cauliflower
Carrots	String beans	Summer squash
Celery	Tomatoes	Eggplant
Green pepper	Zucchini	Turnips

Fruits
One serving equals 40 calories of fresh, frozen or canned without sugar.

If packed in concentrated fruit juice, omit the juice. Frozen juices usually do not contain sugar, but read label to check.

Apples 1 small
Apple juice ⅓ cup
Applesauce (unsweetened) ½ cup
Apricots, fresh 2 med
Apricots, dried 4 halves
Bananas ½ small
Berries
    ½ cup of blackberries, blueberries, raspberries
    ¾ cup of strawberries
Cherries 10 large
Cider ⅓ cup
Dates 2
Figs, fresh 1
Figs, dried 1
Grapefruit ½
Grapefruit juice ½ cup
Grapes 12
Grape juice ½ cup
Mangoes ½ small
Melons
    Cantaloupe ¼ small
    Honeydew ⅛ med
    Watermelon 1 cup

Oranges 1 small
Orange juice ½cup

Papayas ¾ cup
Peaches 1 med
Pear 1 small
Persimmon 1 med

Pineapples ½ cup
Pineapple juice ⅓ cup
Plums 2 med
Prunes 2 med
Prune juice ¼ cup
Raisins 2 tbsp
Tangerines 1 med
Nectarines 1 small
Cranberries — no limit if no
    sugar added.

Complex Carbohydrates

Whole grain breads and cereals
Pita bread
Pastas (avoid those made from white flour;
try whole-wheat or spinach noodles)
Brown rice
Barley Bulgur
Legumes: lentils, beans, peas
Millet
Oats
Wheat germ

Dairy products (limit to two servings a day)
>Eggs
>Fleishman's Egg Beaters (low-cholesterol egg substitute)
>Skim milk
>Buttermilk
>Low-fat yoghurt
>Skim-milk cheeses
>Farmer's cheese
>Cottage cheese

Fish

Almost all fresh and frozen fish are acceptable; avoid salted and pickled fish and those packed in brine or oil. Choose instead canned tuna and salmon packed in water with reduced salt. Shellfish are high in sodium but low in fat; women with problems with fluid retention may want to limit these items.

Blue fish	Clams
Flounder	Lobster
Halibut	Oysters
Monk fish	Scallops
Salmon	Shrimp
Sea bass	
Snapper	
Sole	
Trout	
Tuna	
Whiting	

Lean Meats

Remove skin from poultry; trim fat from meats. Broil, bake or boil; do not fry. Do not use fats in cooking.
>Turkey
>Chicken
>Cornish game hen
>Veal
>Limit intake of beef, lamb and pork

Vegetables (Starchy, eat in moderation)
>Corn

Lima beans
Parsnips
Frozen peas
Potatoes
Pumpkin
Winter squash

Good snack foods are:

Apple, orange and grapefruit juice
Bananas or any fruit on above list
Melba toast
Matzoh
Unsalted pretzels
Unsalted, unbuttered popcorn
Zwieback toast
Unsalted whole wheat crackers
Arrowroot cookies
Ginger snaps
Vanilla wafers
Lorna Doones
Angel food cake, without icing
Graham crackers

Chapter 23

> *"Our studies at Harvard suggest that the average physician knows a little more about nutrition than the average secretary unless the secretary has a weight problem. Then she probably knows more than the average physician."*
>
> Jean Mayer, M.D.

Vitamin Therapy

Women with premenstrual syndrome, like runners preparing for the Boston marathon, need to take all the preventive measures they can to fight the stress and physical effects of their symptoms. They can ill afford the luxury of imbalanced diets or vitamin deficiencies. We recommend that our patients adopt a daily vitamin and mineral supplement as part of the overall lifestyle program. It's especially important for women with poor nutritional habits because dietary changes can't be accomplished overnight. For women with mild to moderate PMS, improved diet, regular exercise, and vitamin supplements may be sufficient to control the illness.

Our own assessments confirm those of other researchers that many women with PMS have faulty eating habits and nutritional deficiencies. If you are able to balance your food intake and achieve the recommended dietary allowances (RDA) recommended by the National Academy of Sciences, you may not need vitamin supplementation. Or you may need only a few months of additional vitamin intake to compensate for your past dietary deficits. We urge you to consult your own physician or a trained nutritionist concerning your specific dietary needs.

At our centers we recommend that women with PMS consume a mid-range of all the important vitamins and minerals over a period of four to eight weeks in order to assess each patient's individual needs and response to these nutrients. Age, weight, height, lifestyle, and health status are contributing factors in determining an individual's nutritional requirements. We use the following range of daily allowances for our patients:

Fat Soluble:

Vitamin A	5,000-12,000 I.U.
D	400-600 I.U.
E	100-300 I.U. Water Soluble (essential):

Water Soluble (essential):

Vitamin C	1,000-3,000 milligrams
Folic Acid	500-1,000 mcg
Thiamine (B_1)	50-150 mg
Riboflavin (B_2)	50-150 mg
Niacin (B_3)	100-300 mg
Pyridoxine (B_6)	100-300 mg
Cobalamin (B_{12})	50-150 mcg
Pantothenic Acid	100-200 mg
Biotin	50-150 mcg

Water Soluble (not established):

Inositol	100-200 mg
PABA	50-150 mg
Pangamate	25-75
Bioflavonoids	50-100 mg

All of the essential B vitamins must be taken together in balanced quantities to be most effective and to avoid aggravating various forms of anemia. The greatest flexibility can be achieved by choosing three separate supplement products — one containing Vitamin C alone, another with the water-soluable vitamins, and a third with the fat-soluble vitamins. Or you may choose a product such as Optivite, which was developed by Dr. Guy Abraham after he undertook research into the nutritional imbalances of women with PMS.

We also emphasize the importance of the B-complex vitamins, particularly B_6.

The B-Complex

The B-complex vitamins — B_1, B_2, B_3, B_6, and B_{12} — are in the starting line-up of the body's essential nutrients. As a team, they play an important role in producing energy, in central nervous system function, in the metabolism of carbohydrates and proteins, and stimulation of the immune response. B_{12}, which contains cobalt, is essential to the formation of the nucleic acids RNA and DNA in the rapid regeneration of bone marrow and the production of red blood cells.

The B-complex vitamins' involvement in premenstrual syndrome was identified more than forty years ago, when some symptoms — nervous tension, anxiety, irritability, and mood swings — were observed in women with B-vitamin deficiencies. But the physician who reported this link noticed marked improvement in his patients after treatment with rice bran extracts and brewer's yeast. Further research revealed that the liver could not deactivate estrogens when a B-vitamin deficiency existed; one theory suggests that an excess of estrogens in some women with PMS is caused by the inability of the liver to deactivate them due to B-vitamin deficiency. This theory meshes with recent findings that elevated blood estrogens in some premenstrual syndrome patients are active estrogens. The liver normally inactivates estrogens and the inactivated estrogens are cleared by the kidney in the urine.

Foods containing the B vitamins include:

B_1, or thiamine, and B_2, or riboflavin — liver and organ meats, pork, brewer's yeast, lean meat, eggs, green leafy vegetables, whole grain breads and cereals, nuts and legumes.

B_3, or niacin — liver and organ meats, fish, tuna, dried peas and beans, whole grains, nuts, eggs.

B_{12} — organ and muscle meats, milk, eggs, brewer's yeast, seafood (especially clams, oysters and shrimp).

Vitamin B_6

Pyridoxine, or Vitamin B_6, eases the symptoms of severe PMS, but it usually does not eradicate them. It takes the edge off irritability and reduces fatigue and depression. It may reduce or eliminate breast swelling and headaches. It's not clear how or why B_6 has these effects. We know that it acts on the central nervous system, which might affect the neurotransmitters dopamine and serotonin in the chain of actions that regulate the production of progesterone and other hormones. It may also aid in the liver's metabolism of estrogen. Some women seem unable to tolerate B_6; they may become nauseated or dizzy with vitamin supplements. This is usually because they've been given too high a dosage. Decreasing the dosage will usually resolve the problem. B_6 and the B-complex supplement should be taken with a meal to increase their absorption. We usually start our patients with 50 milligrams of B_6 and slowly build up to 200 to 500 mg.

B_6 might be viewed as the most valuable player of the B-complex, a critical component in growth, repair of cells, and the production of energy. It aids in the breakdown of the body's building blocks, amino acids, from ingested proteins, their synthesis from compounds within the body, their subsequent absorption into the cells, and their eventual formation into proteins. It also acts as a co-enzyme in the formation of hemoglobin, the protein that carries oxygen from the lungs to each of the cells. (Hemoglobin circulates in the bloodstream). Pyridoxine also is active in the metabolism of fats and carbohydrates. Without B_6 the body's cells could not produce energy.

A deficiency of B_6 first affects the nervous system, especially in children; in adults, especially women, it may be manifested as depression. This is because the brain needs proteins to function and with a B_6 deficiency the protein supply to the brain is greatly reduced. Since B_6 is involved in the metabolism of amino acids, as well as in the formation of the substance that holds them together — collagen — a deficiency not only interferes with repairs and growth but can result in serious structural damage to the gums, teeth, bones, and liver, and lowered immune response.

B_6 deficiency is not common, in part because the vitamin is stable to heat and acid; it's more resistant to food processing and storage than other vitamins and minerals. Adequate amounts of B_6 are usually obtained in a normal diet. Women taking oral contraceptives, however, commonly have B_6 deficiencies, marked by depression. Not all women become depressed when using oral contraceptives. And of those who do, not all depression is necessarily due to pyridoxine deficiency. But among women on the pill who also have a B_6 deficiency, B_6 supplements can usually eliminate the depression. Some researchers have concluded that women with a history of depression, premenstrual depression, or depression during pregnancy — and who become worse after starting the pill — are most likely to respond to pyridoxine. In one study, two hundred twenty out of two hundred fifty women responded to pyridoxine therapy for their depression. Oral contraceptives also interfere with the body's ability to metabolize carbohydrates and remove them from the bloodstream for storage in the liver. In some women, this side effect can reach a state similar to that of diabetes. Supplements of B_6 help restore the glucose metabolism to a more normal range.

B_6 has also been found to alleviate nausea and discomfort in pregnant women, and it plays a role in fertility. Large doses of B_6 suppress the secretion of prolactin, a hormone which stimulates lactation and inhibits conception, thus preventing pregnancy. This is one of the body's protective devices to prevent pregnancy in a woman who's already pregnant or breast-feeding. Dr. Guy Abraham has shown that when a group of fourteen infertile women with premenstrual tension were given supplements of pyridoxine, ranging from 100 to 800 mg, for at least six months, twelve of them suddenly became fertile and conceived.

Nutritional sources of pyridoxine are liver and organ meats, whole grain cereals and bread, wheat germ, soybeans, brewer's yeast, nuts, red meat, fish, spinach, avocados, bananas, green beans, green leafy vegetables, potatoes, molasses, cabbage, and green peppers. Vegetables should be eaten raw because cooking destroys the vitamin.

Pyridoxine is available in supplements ranging from 5 to 500 milligrams; most over-the-counter vitamin supplements include 2 mg of B_6, the recommended daily allowance. There is no known toxicity of large doses of B_6; although it has been suggested by researchers that doses exceeding two grams per day may cause peripheral nerve damage. Overdoses from the normal diet are all but impossible.

Optivite, the supplement developed by Dr. Abraham, is available from Optimox Inc., P.O. Box 7000-280, Rolling Hills Estates, CA. 90274.

Chapter 24

"The wise, for cure, on exercise depend."

John Dryden, *Epistle*
to John Driden of Chesterton

Getting Physical

Regular exercise is another important weapon in the anti-PMS arsenal. It ameliorates the symptoms of depression, anxiety, fatigue, irritability, nervous energy, premenstrual headaches, and cramps. Depression is especially helped by regular exercise; studies have shown that the improvement in the efficiency of the cardiovascular and respiratory systems by aerobic exercise speeds recovery from depression. The patients we see who begin a regular exercise program do report a lessening of the severity of their PMS symptoms. Women with mild to moderate cases may find that exercise and nutritional changes may be sufficient therapy, either to eliminate the symptoms completely, or to reduce them to a minor inconvenience. Many women find that exercise alone is not enough; some must also adhere to a dietary program to gain relief. We put all of our patients at the center on an exercise program because we believe that PMS treatment requires a combination of therapy: diet, exercise, and stress management are essential. In many cases, vitamin supplements are called for; severe cases of PMS, of course, will also require progesterone therapy.

Why does exercise help? It speeds up weight loss on any type of diet. It improves circulatory and oxygenating capacity. It may also increase the secretion of progesterone and beta-endorphins, the hormones that are released by the brain and produce a sensation of mild euphoria.

We strongly advise women, whether or not they have PMS, to begin and continue an exercise routine. By regular, we mean three times a week for a minimum of fifteen to thirty minutes each time. Fifteen minutes of vigorous exercise are required to boost your heart rate and increase its efficiency. No more than two days should elapse between workouts or the gains made on Monday will be lost by Wednesday night.

Before undertaking any exercise program, however, make sure to:

1. *Consult a physician*. Make sure you are in good health and can undertake a program without potential problems. A physician can identify any medical problems you might have, point out your limitations and suggest suitable forms of exercise that will not jeopardize your health.

2. *Choose appropriate clothing*. Wear warm, comfortable, and loose-fitting clothing. It is better to be overdressed than underdressed. On cooler days muscles take longer to warm up and relax. To avoid tears and strains of muscles you need extra protection. Proper footwear protects the sensitive bones and muscle in the feet and legs. A structured bra gives extra support to the breasts.

3. *Begin a regimen slowly and carefully*. Always warm up slowly before beginning calisthenics or any athletic activity. Don't push yourself beyond your limits initially. Your body will tell you when to stop. Exercise should stretch and flex your muscles, not cause pain. If you feel pain, stop. Aches and stiffness, however, are the natural byproducts of a new exercise regime. A long soak in a hot tub, sauna, or jacuzzi will turn that stiffness into a memory.

One way to determine if you're in good condition is the pinch test for body fat. Extend your arm away from your body so that the upper arm is level with your shoulder and bend your elbow slightly to make a muscle. With the thumb and forefinger of the other hand, pinch the skin on the back of the raised arm over your triceps muscle in the middle of your under-upper-arm. The pinch should be made lengthwise. Estimate the amount of skin and fat you could pinch, or have a friend measure it with a ruler. The average amount of skin and fat a physically fit person has is one-half to three-quarter inches. If you have less than one-quarter of inch of skin and fat, you have a very low body fat level and are probably in better-than-average shape. If you have more than three-quarters of an inch, you've got a lot of work to do to get in shape.

If you're already an active woman of normal weight who follows some kind of exercise program, you should be able to complete the following calisthenics regime quickly and advance to more intensive aerobic exercises, like aerobic dancing, swimming, running, bicycling or other sports. If, however, you are out of shape, overweight, or haven't been exercising regularly, you'll have to take it slow at first. Here's how to start:

Warm Ups: Relaxation and Breathing Exercises

1. Reach both hands over your head, stand on tiptoe and stretch, breathing in very slowly and deeply. While breathing out, gently fold at the waist and try to touch your toes with your fingertips. Do not strain yourself doing this. Repeat this exercise six times with a stretch and inhale up, and relax and exhale down.

2. While standing with your feet apart, extend one arm loosely above your head with the other at your side. Bend slowly six times to the side opposite your extended arm. Then reverse the position of your arms and bend six times to the other side. Be certain to come up fully to the upright position after each repetition.

3. Sit down comfortably on the floor with your legs extended straight in front of you and slightly apart. Stretch as far as you can toward your toes without pain, come back up to the upright position and stretch your arms over your head and down to your toes again. Remember, inhale up, exhale down. Six repetitions.

4. Lie flat on the floor, legs stretched out straight in front of you. Raise one leg. Using your hands, pull your knee toward your chest. Return to the original prone position. Repeat six times with each leg.

5. Remain in the prone position, arms extended flat on the floor at the shoulder level. Slowly bend your legs and bring your knees up to your chest. Keeping your knees together, roll slowly to one side until the outside knee touches the floor. Then roll to the other side and touch the other knee to the floor. Six repetitions.

Walking

After completing the warm-up exercises, it's time to go outside for a brisk walk. Remember to breath deeply and slowly as you walk. Start out slowly with a walk around the block the first day. Over a two-week period, increase the distance of your walk to a mile. Increase your walking distance and speed as you desire and feel comfortable. Try to walk at least one mile briskly each day five days a week.

Those who choose walking as their primary exercise should slowly but surely increase the distance of the walk, but decrease the amount of time it takes to cover.

A good progression, to be covered five times a week, is:

WEEK 1	1 mile in 15 minutes.
WEEK 2	1 mile in 14 minutes.
WEEK 3	1 mile in 13 minutes and 45 seconds.
WEEK 4	1½ in 21 minutes and 30 seconds.
WEEK 5	1½ in 21 minutes.
WEEK 6	1½ in 20 minutes and 30 seconds.
WEEK 7	2 miles in 28 minutes.
WEEK 8	2 miles in 27 minutes and 45 seconds.
WEEK 9	2 miles in 27 minutes and 30 seconds.

The routine is varied from this point on:

WEEK 10   2 miles in 27 minutes and 30 seconds three times a week and 2½ miles in 35 minutes and 30 seconds twice a week.

WEEK 11   2 miles in 27 minutes and 30 seconds three times a week and 2½ miles in 35 minutes twice a week.

WEEK 12   2½ miles in 34 minutes and 30 seconds four times a week and 3 miles in 41 minutes and 30 seconds once.

WEEK 13   2½ miles in 33 minutes and 15 seconds three times a week and 3 miles in 42 minutes twice a week.

WEEK 14   2½ miles in 33 minutes three times a week and 3 miles in 41 minutes and 30 seconds twice a week.

WEEK 15   3 miles in 42 minutes five times a week.

WEEK 16   4 miles in 56 minutes four times a week.

Calisthenics

For those who prefer calisthenics as their primary form of exercise, we recommend following the first two weeks of the walking program to ease yourself into a routine. Walking is an excellent base for any exercise program. We encourage our patients to walk a mile a day briskly before undertaking any other exercise. Once you've reached that one mile walking goal, you're ready to try calisthenics.

From the following exercises, choose two to three exercises from each category and do them at least three times a week. And remember: Relax, breath deeply and slowly, and enjoy yourself.

Moderate.

Stand upright, feet planted widely, arms extended straight overhead and hands clasped. Bend your knees slightly and fold forward at the waist, keeping your head between your arms. Circle at the waist four times clockwise and four times counterclockwise, raising your head and arms slowly as you progress, until you are upright with head and hands extending toward the ceiling. Repeat six times. Remember to breath deeply as you exercise.

Moderate.

This exercise requires an object that weighs about two pounds, a household item, like an iron or can of fruits or vegetables. Stand with feet wide apart, arms at side. Hold the weight in one hand at the side of your body. Bend side to side, dropping your head with your body as you bend. Repeat ten times.

Moderate.

Sit comfortably on the floor with feet wide apart, arms extended at shoulder level, straight out to the sides. Bend your body slightly forward and twist it gently at the waist to touch your right hand to your left foot. Repeat with left hand to right foot. Return to upright position. Repeat ten times.

Moderate.

Kneel on the floor. Extend one leg straight out to the side, with arms straight out overhead, hands clasped. Bend sideways over the outstretched leg. Keep looking forward. Take ten bends to one side. Then switch and extend the opposite leg and complete ten repetitions to the other side.

Advanced.

Lie on the floor, legs wide apart. Extend arms straight overhead with hands clasped. Do a full situp. With arms still straight overhead, stretch twice toward your left foot, stretching as far as comfortably as possible. Return to upright position. Repeat twice toward right foot, and then twice toward the space between your feet. Lie back down in prone position. Repeat this eight times.

For the Arms

Moderate.
Hold your two-pound weight in one hand with an underhand grip.
Keeping your elbow at your side, flex your elbow and raise the weight to
chest level. Then lower it. Repeat with each arm ten times.

Moderate.
Stand with legs apart, knees slightly bent, bending forward at the
waist, arms at your sides. Swing one arm forward and the other
backward. Repeat ten times. Then hold arms straight out at sides for a
slow count of twenty.

Moderate.
Lie down on your back on the floor. Take your two-pound weight in
your right hand and rest it on the floor beside you. Supporting your
upper right arm with your left hand, extend your elbow and lift the
weight with a straight right arm toward the ceiling slowly. Return to
original position. Repeat with each arm ten times.

Advanced.
Stand facing a wall, hands in front of you braced against the wall
extended at shoulder level. Lean into the wall, bending your elbows
toward the floor. Straighten your arms and push yourself away from the
wall. Be sure to keep your back straight and breathe deeply. To increase
the difficulty of the exercise, increase your distance from the wall. Eight
repetitions.

Advanced.
Stand with legs apart, knees slightly bent, bending forward at the
waist, arms at your side. Take two two-pound weights in each hand.
Swing one arm forward and the other backward. Repeat ten times. Then
hold arms straight out at sides for a slow count of twenty.

For the Abdomen

Moderate.
Lie flat on your back on the floor, arms extended straight overhead.
With one knee bent, one leg out straight, bring outstretched leg straight

up halfway. Then bring top half of body up to meet the leg in the middle. Hold for a count of five. Relax and repeat eight times for each leg.

Moderate.

Lie on your back on the floor with hands clasped behind your head. Legs should extend straight out. Lift your head and upper body as you tuck your right knee to your chest. Touch your left elbow to the right knee and return to beginning position. Repeat with right elbow and left knee. Eight repetitions.

Moderate.

Lie on your back with your hands under your buttocks to flatten the arch in your back. Tuck your knees into your chest. Extend legs straight in the air. Tuck them back to your chest. Extend legs straight out on floor. Eight times.

Advanced.

Sit on the floor with your feet tucked under the edge of a heavy chair or courch. Lie flat on the floor with knees bent and arms extended straight overhead. Move your buttocks as close to your feet as is comfortably possible. Try to keep your biceps at ear level and chin tucked into your chest as you crawl up and touch your knees. Inhale as you lower your body and exhale as you sit up. Eight repetitions.

Advanced.

Lie on the floor on your back, resting your weight on your elbows with legs extended straight. Push up elbows and tuck knees into chest simultaneously. Move as far as possible with feet off floor. Return to original position. Eight times.

Bust

Moderate

Clasp right wrist with left hand, left wrist with right hand directly in front of your chest. Grip securely and push one arm against the other. Hold for a count of five and release. Eight times.

Moderate

Sit comfortably and clasp your hands behind your head. Pull your elbows back so your shoulder blades come together. Hold for a count of five. Repeat five times.

Moderate

Lie face down, elbows to the side, hands clasped, palms on the floor. Rest your forehead on your hands. Lift head, hands and elbows two inches from the floor. Hold for count of five. Eight times.

Hips, Buttocks

Moderate

Lie on the floor on your side. Support your head with your hand. Lift your upper leg, straight up, with toe pointing. Eight times. Roll over and repeat eight times with other leg.

Moderate

On your hands and knees, extend one leg out to the side, raise leg and lower. Repeat ten times with each leg.

Moderate

Lie face down on the floor, hands clasped in front of you with chin resting on the back of your hands. Slowly lift one leg straight up and hold for a count of five. Relax. Repeat six times with each leg.

Moderate

Stand up straight. With arm extended to your side at shoulder level, grasp the back of a chair. Lift outside leg and make ten large, slow circles. Repeat with other leg.

Moderate

Still holding on to the chair, lift outside leg forward, to the side, and back ten times. Repeat with other leg.

Moderate

Sitting on the floor, one leg out straight and the other leg with knee bent and foot against the inside of the opposite knee. Keep your hands resting on the floor. Bring your bent knee to touch the floor on both sides, going back and forth. Ten times.

Moderate

Lie on your back with your hands under your buttocks to support your back. Lift your legs and pedal as if you were riding a bicycle. Count to thirty slowly. Rest and repeat.

Moderate

Stand up straight, feet widely planted. Hold a pole or broom handle, palms down. Lift the pole straight overhead, inhale deeply. Exhale as you bend your elbows and lower the pole behind your back. Inhale as you extend the pole over your head and exhale as you return it to the original position. Six times.

Moderate

Stand straight up with feet widely planted, hold the pole or broom overhead with arms fully extended. Bend your knees slightly and lean from side to side at the waist slowly in a continuous motion. Eight times.

Advanced

Lie on your side with your body straight and your head resting on your hand. Lift both legs lightly off the floor with top leg slightly off bottom leg. Kick in a scissor fashion for thirty seconds. Roll over and repeat on the other side.

Advanced

On your hands and knees, tuck one knee into chest and tuck head down as close to knee as possible. Lift your head and extend leg straight out behind you. Repeat ten times with each leg.

Advanced

On hands and knees, extend one leg straight out to your side. Lift it as high as is comfortable to the side. Swing it directly in back of you and lift. Repeat six times with each leg.

After completing the basic beginner's calisthenics program, you may want to advance to a more strenuous exercise regimen. We recommend aerobic exercise as a supplement to any good fitness program because it increases cardiovascular respiratory efficiency and strength and flexibility of the large muscles of the body. The best aerobic exercises are aerobic dancing, bicycle riding, swimming, jogging, and running. Remember that to bring any health benefits, a program must be undertaken at least three times a week for a minimum of twenty minutes of strenuous activity.

How can you tell if an exercise is aerobic? The exercise should increase cardiopulmonary fitness, and condition muscles but not strain them. The program should help you reach a "target zone" of sixty to eighty percent of your maximum attainable pulse rate. Generally this maximum attainable rate is determined by subtracting your age from the number 220. Sixty to eighty percent of that figure is your target zone. (If you're thirty years old, your target zone is 114 to 152 beats a minute, or sixty to eighty percent of 190.)

To test yourself, pause at intervals during your workout and take your pulse. In taking your pulse at your wrist, never use the thumb because it has a pulse of its own. Instead, use the second and third fingers, placing them along the inside or thumb side of your wrist. Press in gently until you feel the beat of the artery. Looking at the second hand of a clock or watch, count the beats in a ten-second time period and multiply by six to determine the rate per minute. An alternative method is to take the pulse of the artery in your neck. Again using the second and third fingers, gently probe down from the jaw bone and push in lightly until you feel the pulse beat. Again, count the beat in a ten-second period and multiple by six.

If you're just beginning an aerobics program, keep your pulse rate down toward the lower limit of the target zone so you won't overtax your heart. As your body condition improves and the cardiorespiratory system strengthens, you should try to approach the upper limit. Remember, keep all your exercise routines at a comfortable and slow pace initially.

Any aerobic regimen should include:

• *A five to ten minute* warmup and moderate aerobic exercises to stimulate the circulatory system and warm up the muscles.

• *A ten to twenty minute* peak period in which you reach and maintain your target zone pulse rate.

• *A five to ten minute* cool down routine of moderate aerobic exercises that permits the blood to return to all parts of the body and not remain trapped in the hands or feet.

An important aspect of any aerobic program is enjoyment. Whatever method of exercise you choose should be something that you can look forward to at least three times a week, week in and week out over a lifetime.

Chapter 25/ *Managing Stress*

Stress is a damaging factor in most of our lives and is an element implicated in all diseases. Like the oily extortionist in a turn-of-the-century melodrama who ties the stubborn heroine onto railroad tracks as a speeding train approaches, stress is the villain pressuring us, threatening our health and emotional stability. In an illness as complex and chronic as premenstrual syndrome, stress adds a dangerous and volatile variable to the scene; it compounds the problems and exacerbates the symptoms of PMS, which itself is a major source of stress. Women with PMS cannot be successfully treated for their illness unless they reduce the stress in their daily routine and learn to manage the stress they can't avoid.

In his book, *The Stress of Life,* the late Dr. Hans Selye explained that stress could be caused by such disparate factors as infection, noise, overcrowding, tumultuous but generally positive events such as vacation, Christmas and other holidays, marriage, or a sudden rise in financial status. The body adapts to these diverse stressors in the same way no matter what the source of the stress or what organ is involved. Selye, who won the Nobel Prize for his identification of what he termed the General Adaptation Syndrome or GAS, identified three stages in the stress syndrome: alarm, resistance, and exhaustion. Each of the stages is associated with specific bodily changes in the same organs.

Stress encompasses any event, whether positive or negative, that forces the body to make an adjustment. To illustrate, if you suffer a minor cut, a localized mechanism called the Local Adaptation Syndrome, or LAS, is activated. LAS is linked, in the case of the cut, to the process of local repair of injured tissues. The GAS and the LAS are closely linked, like the command and operating units of fire and police departments. The GAS is the command unit, answering the body's stress symptoms as if they were a call to 911. LAS is the on-the-scene emergency crew, the engine crew or police squad sent off to report on and repair the damage. Both set off identical physical defenses in the body. Both involve the release of a pituitary hormone that stimulates the adrenal gland to secrete the hormones necessary for the defense or repair of the body. The physical changes that result from stress are the body's attempt to somehow adapt to the cause of stress, be it noise, grief, or extreme cold. Our bodies pay as high a toll for emotional stress as they do for physical stress, especially if it's chronic, because the changes brought on by either are identical.

The three stages of stress are actual physiological events, but psychological factors play an important part in the way the body copes with stress. As Dr. Jay M. Weiss of the Rockefeller University, a leader in stress disease research, says the more helpless one feels in a situation, the more likely one is to develop a stress-related disease. The secret of remaining calm is a great one to master, but it isn't simply a matter of repressing feelings of anger or fear triggered by stress.

How the Body Deals With Stress

The hypothalamus and the pituitary, both of which orchestrate the production of sex hormones, also orchestrate the body's response to stress. When the alarm stage of stress is triggered, the hypothalamus sends frantic hormonal messages to the pituitary gland. That signal means the body needs energy to cope with a physical emergency. This is most commonly known as the fight or flight response. The pituitary, as soon as it receives the hypothalamus's message, sends out a hormone called ACTH. ACTH goes to a part of the adrenal gland known as the adrenal cortex. It acts exclusively on the adrenal cortex, which finds its home wrapped around the adrenal gland above each kidney. The triggering of the fight-or-flight hormone increases the blood sugar level, while pupils dilate, muscles contract, and blood pressure rises temporarily. The body prepares to make a stand. As a kind of contingency action, it also releases certain substances which aid the cells in repairing themselves. These substances released by the adrenal gland include one most closely linked with feelings of anger and tension: norepinephrine, which is secreted by the inner portion of the adrenal, the medulla. This stimulates the central nervous system, an experience we undergo when we are angry. An injection of norepinephrine into the brain will cause anyone to feel anger, no matter how peaceful they were the moment preceding the injection. Individuals who secrete this substance in excess will feel tense and angry a lot of the time. Norepinephrine constricts the blood vessels; it also acts in conjunction with another hormone from the

adrenal cortex, aldosterone, to raise one's blood pressure. The activation of the response in a person with a high sodium intake can turn
anxiety into a very real and deadly physical malady. In today's world,
most people have little opportunity to vent their emotions or act out the
fight/flight response. As a result, the hormones keep the body in a state
of constant preparation for battles that are never fought. The resultant
tension without release changes the body's response to excess sodium,
making it more easily retained.

With aldosterone acting to retain salt and fluids and norepinephrine
constricting the blood vessels, the result is high blood pressure. The
increase in blood pressure, when triggered by stress, lasts as long as the
stress lasts. In major stress, the body reaches the stage of exhaustion.

Stress leaves scars on the internal organs, especially on the adrenal
glands. Dr. Selye was fond of noting that no one dies of old age, they
just lose their ability to adapt to stress. Instead of bending, they break.
To prevent the breaks and teach individuals how to bend, several stress
evaluation systems and a score of stress management techniques have
been developed over the past two decades, including biofeedback and
the relaxation response program of Dr. Herbert Benson of the Harvard
Medical School and Beth Israel Hospital in Boston. A classic stress
measurement test was developed in 1967 by Thomas Holmes and
Richard Rahe, psychiatrists at the University of Washington School of
Medicine. Their barometer, which they call the Social Readjustment
Scale, rates the stressfulness of various life events from little stress (1)
to most stressful (100). Review the items and check off those that you
have experienced within the previous twelve months. If your score
reaches or exceeds 300, you're over-stressed and have a 90 percent
chance of becoming ill or having a major accident because of stress.

Social Readjustment Scale

Death of spouse	100
Divorce	73
Marital separation	65
Incarceration (prison term)	63
Death of immediate family member	63
Personal injury or illness	53
Marriage	50
Discharged from job	47

Marital reconciliation	4
Retirement	4
Change in health of family member	4
Pregnancy	4
Sexual problems	3
Gain of new family member	3
Business readjustment	3
Change in financial status	3
Death of a close friend	3
Change of careers	3
Change in number of arguments with mate	3
Mortgage over $10,000	3
Foreclosure of debt	3
Change in job responsibilities	2
Child leaving home	2
Trouble with in-laws	2
Outstanding personal achievement	2
Begin or end of school	2
Spouse begins or stops work	2
Change in living conditions	2
Change in personal habits	2
Conflicts with employer or supervisor	2
Change in work hours or conditions	2
Change of residence	2
Change of schools	2
Change in recreation	1
Change in church activities	1
Change in social activities	1
Mortgage or loan less than $10,000	1
Change in sleeping habits	1
Change in eating habits	1
Vacation	1
Christmas	1
Minor violations of law	1

Adapting this social stress measure to women with premenstrual syndrome, we ask our patients to indicate what stress indicators they may have experienced in the past two years and within the past twelve months to determine how stressful their lives are, what role stress may be playing in adding to or exacerbating the PMS symptoms, and to identify and help them reduce specific stressors. The questionnaire we use follows. Look it over. How many of these stressors are present or

Life Events

The following checklist consists of events which are sometimes important experiences. Please read down the list until you find events that have happened to you personally. Then indicate two things:

When did the event occur? Check "Time Period"

Do you still think about the event? Often, At Times, No?

Life Event	Time Period		Still Think About It		
	Within past 2 years	More than 2 years	Often	At Times	No
Death of Spouse					
Divorce					
Marital separation					
Jail term					
Death of a close family member					
Personal injury or illness					
Marriage					
Fired at work					
Marital reconciliation or serious problem					
Retirement					
Change in health of family member ...					
Pregnancy					
Sex difficulties					
Gain of a new family member					
Business readjustment					
Change in financial state					
Death of a close friend					
Change to different line of work					
Change in number of arguments with spouse					
Mortgage over $50,000					
Foreclosure of mortgage or loan					
Change in responsibilities at work					
Son or daughter leaving home					
Trouble with in-laws					
Outstanding personal achievement					
Spouse begins or stops work					

Life Event	Time Period		Still Think About It		
	Within past 2 years	More than 2 years	Often	At Times	No
Begin or end school					
Change in living conditions					
Revision of personal habits					
Trouble with boss					
Change in work hours or conditions ..					
Change in residence					
Change in schools					
Change in recreation					
Change in church activities					
Change in social activities					
Mortgage or loan less than $50,000					
Change in sleeping habits					
Change in number of family get-togethers					
Change in eating habits					
Vacation					
Christmas					
Minor violation of the law					

have been present recently in your life? To accommodate the inflationary spiral of housing costs, you'll note that we have pegged our mortgage and loan levels to $50,000, instead of the $10,000 used by Holmes and Rahe in 1967.

Relaxation Techniques

Any number of methods of relaxation can be used to slow the heart rate and lower blood pressure: relaxation response, meditation, deep breathing exercises, yoga, biofeedback, cognitive training. If you have tried any of these techniques and found they work for you, continue to use them. Two basic methods to divert your mind from stress that can be used twice a day, or whenever you're in a stressful situation, involve breathing and muscle exercises. Both of them can be done at your desk, at home, in connection with other exercises, or even in bed if you have trouble falling asleep.

Breathing Exercise

Sit back in a comfortable chair, feet flat on the floor, arms loose. Close your eyes, relax all your muscles, starting from the feet up, calves, thighs, abdomen, arms. Loosen up your shoulders, head, and neck. Sit quietly, breathe very slowly and naturally. Try to clear your mind. Choose a word or number that you will focus on repeatedly during the exercise. Those who meditate or use yoga may already have a mantra, or single syllable upon which they concentrate as they try to empty their mind of diversionary thoughts. If you have a mantra, use it during this exercise. As you breath slowly and quietly, say the word or number to yourself as you exhale. At each exhalation, repeat the word to yourself. Other thoughts may intrude, but let them pass. Don't get annoyed at that or focus on it. Just keep breathing slowly, and as you exhale, repeat your chosen word to yourself. Let's say your word is love. Breath slowly and deeply, and as you exhale repeat the word love to yourself. Inhale, exhale while thinking of the word love. Inhale, exhale, repeating love. Do this for several minutes. Keep your eyes closed, but slowly begin to let your mind focus on normal thoughts. Then very slowly open your eyes.

This is a good exercise to do twice a day for 10 to 20 minutes, to clear your mind and force yourself to slow down. You might find it easy to adopt this method into your daily routine immediately, but most people find that it takes several days for them to be able to handle a 10- to 20-minute session.

Muscle Relaxation

Sit in a comfortable chair, in a comfortable position, both feet on the floor, arms loose.

Focus on your toes. Think about them. Then tighten up your toes, hold that position for a count of three, and release.

Next focus on your calves. Tighten the calf muscles, hold the pose for a count of three, and release.

Then the thighs. Tighten the top muscles of the thighs, hold it for three seconds, and release.

Continue this progressive concentration on the major muscle groups of the body: buttocks and abdomen, small of back and waist, upper body, chest and back.

Now make your hands into fists. Clench them tightly, count to three and release.

Then try to tense your lower arms, the upper arms and biceps, shoulders and neck muscles, and finally, the face. Grimace as tightly as you can to contract the face muscles, hold it for a count of three, and release.

If after finishing this routine you feel that a part of your body is still gripped in tension, repeat the routine for that muscle group. This is a good exercise to adopt two or three times a day.

Chapter 26

*"Science is a first-rate piece
of furniture for a man's upper
chamber, if he has common sense
on the ground floor."*

Oliver Wendell Holmes, **The Poet
at the Breakfast Table**

The Progesterone Story

For women with chronic cases of premenstrual syndrome the search for treatment has most likely resembled an odyssey with many more than twelve obstacles blocking the way. The frustration and anger that mounts each time a promised "cure" fails feeds a relentless need. By the time they come to us for treatment many women are looking for a miracle. Progesterone is not a miracle cure, not a magic bullet. It is simply the most effective treatment known for premenstrual syndrome. For most of the women we have treated, it has eliminated or sharply reduced the symptoms. But progesterone cannot work miracles; and it does not produce the best results unless it is used in conjunction with the lifestyle changes discussed in earlier chapters.

The results of progesterone therapy are impressive. In examining the treatment results of a small sample of our patients — one hundred women treated at our clinic for six to fourteen months — seventy-seven of the women were symptom-free at the time of the survey. Twenty-three patients were significantly improved: most of their symptoms had abated, but one symptom remained (usually headaches). But it, too, was less frequent and/or less intense. Five patients no longer required progesterone because their symptoms had remitted. Each patient had a severe case of PMS with multiple symptoms that had been present for more than five years; each woman had made at least three prior attempts at treatment for PMS without success. None of these patients had ever had a term pregnancy, i.e. actually delivered a child.

We don't know yet precisely how or why progesterone alleviates the wide-ranging symptoms of premenstrual syndrome. Medical science must first identify the scope of the role of progesterone and estrogen in the body, and research must be done to pinpoint the cause or causes of premenstrual syndrome. Progesterone does have analgesic and sedative properties; it makes you feel good. Some physicians say that the analgesic effect is what eases the complaints of many women. The complexity of PMS and its range of symptoms indicate, however, that the disorder is too complicated to be put to rest by a sedative and that progesterone plays a critical role in an intricate hormonal balance that is somehow disturbed, producing PMS.

Before we go any further, you need to master the vocabulary we'll be using:

Progestational agents — substances, either produced by the body or compounded synthetically, that act to stimulate uterine changes essential to pregnancy. Progestational means favoring pregnancy, conducive to gestation.

Progestin — a generic term for any substance, natural or synthetic, that has some of the properties of progesterone. The word is used interchangeably with progestogen.

Progestogen — any substance that acts to stimulate uterine changes essential to pregnancy. Progesterone is a progestogen. Only two progestogens occur naturally in the human body: progesterone and 17- alpha-hydroxyprogesterone. All other progestogens are synthetically produced. There are structural molecular differences between these various progestogens, which are reflected in their function within the multiple biological systems in the body and the effects they produce.

Progesterone — the female sex hormone produced primarily by the ovaries during the reproductive years to prepare a woman's body for pregnancy. A molecularly identical compound to naturally occuring progesterone produced by pharmacists is available in injectable or suppository form and is used in the treatment of women with severe cases of premenstrual syndrome. It is this molecularly identical compound we refer to when we use the word "progesterone." Progesterone is both a progestogen and a progestin, but many substances that are progestogens and progestins are not progesterone.

Provera — a prescription drug brand name for a compound of medroxyprogesterone, a synthetic progestogen. It is a compound related to, but distinguishable from, progesterone, and its properties are very different. Physicians all too often confuse Provera with progesterone.

Steroid hormone — substances derived from cholesterol involving a distinctive ring-like chemical structure. The sex hormones — progesterone, estrogen, testosterone, and the corticosteroids — are steroid hormones.

Confusion Over Substances

Many physicians confuse progesterone with other progestational substances, natural or synthetic; they speak of these substances as if they had the same properties and they prescribe them for their patients as if they had the same properties. Progesterone and only progesterone as it naturally occurs in the body is the appropriate therapy for premenstrual syndrome. Many progestogens have properties that antagonize and worsen premenstrual syndrome. Sometimes, to make the distinction between progesterone and progestogens more clear, we emphasize to our patients that progesterone is a naturally occuring substance and that the other progestogens are not. Hence, some women refer to "natural progesterone" vs. "synthetic." This is not precisely accurate, of course. Any substance manufactured in a laboratory is synthetic, including the progesterone suppositories or liquid injectable forms used in this country. But these progesterone compounds are molecular twins of progesterone as it is produced by the ovaries. Progestogens, like Provera and those contained in birth control pills, are made of compounds similar to progesterone, except for subtle differences in molecular structure. It is that subtle difference that can mean pain or relief to a woman with premenstrual syndrome. And it is that subtle difference that many physicians refuse to recognize or do not have the sophistication and training in steroid chemistry to understand.

Progesterone was first used successfully for the treatment of premenstrual syndrome in 1934, the year it was first isolated by Dr. Willard Allen, among others. Since then, a number of researchers have reported its successful use. The rationale for its use was first published by Leon Israel in 1938 who suggested that an uncontrolled estrogen effect resulting from a deficiency of progesterone was the cause of the symptoms. A relative progesterone deficiency in relationship to a possible estrogen excess was subsequently documented in studies of luteal phase steroid levels in women suffering from PMS.

Another documented consequence of deficient luteal phase progesterone levels is the defect which results in an apparent under-development of the lining of the uterus, the endometrium. The endometrium does not develop sufficiently to sustain the implantation of a fertilized egg. Often this is attributed to insufficient progesterone production by the corpus luteum. Miscarriages will result and, in some women, infertility. Luteal phase deficiency occurs in about three percent of the female population, but it has been found in thirty-five to fifty percent of women who suffer from repeated spontaneous abortions and miscarriages. Infertility and miscarriages due to luteal phase defects have been successfully treated with progesterone suppositories. Unless there is an underlying disorder, such as hypothyroidism, the deficiency can be treated with progesterone, usually 25 milligrams twice a day beginning three to four days before the onset of the luteal phase and continuing until the onset of menstruation.

There are no reported significant side effects of progesterone, no adverse interaction between progesterone and other drugs has been documented, and it would be almost impossible to overdose on it. The female body produces ten to thirty times more progesterone in the second and third trimesters of pregnancy than in the peak level of the luteal phase. As Dr. Charles Lloyd, a prominent endocrinologist and former director of the Worcester Foundation for Experimental Biology, where oral contraceptives were first developed, says: "If I were looking for an innocuous substance to take, it would be progesterone. There are no side effects, except in some, a cutting down of the sex drive."

In our clinical experience, peak blood levels of women being treated with progesterone have not approached the blood levels observed in the late second and third trimesters of pregnancy. Probably the only means by which a woman could overdose on progesterone is by intravenous administration. Occasionally, in women who have never carried a child to term and thus have not been exposed to the large amounts of progesterone usually present during pregnancy, progesterone doses by suppository exceeding 400 milligrams may produce mild euphoria, restless energy, faintness, and some uterine cramping.

Studies of the side effects of the long-term use of progesterone have not been completed. Dr. Katharina Dalton has followed many women who have been on continuous progesterone therapy for over ten years and has reported no adverse effects. She has also begun reviewing the medical records of her patients of the last thirty-five years; her results are eagerly awaited. However, these earliest patients of Dr. Dalton who took progesterone for many years need to be assessed in a well-designed epidemiological study to determine if there are possible adverse, or perhaps protective, side effects from the long-term use of progesterone.

No Side-Effects Reported

Progesterone has been administered intravenously over many days continuously in doses of 100 to 150 mg per day without apparent adverse effect and with minimal toxic symptoms. In some published studies, progesterone administered in 500-mg doses intravenously and in several thousand-milligram doses over several days by injection produced no apparent adverse effects and minimal toxic symptoms. Progesterone administered intravenously or by injection reaches the bloodstream directly, so the dosages are lower than those in suppository form. By the suppository method, progesterone is absorbed through the mucus membranes of the vagina or rectum and taken into the system; not all of the progesterone may be absorbed from the suppository and some of its strength and effectiveness is lost in the absorption process. And women metabolize progesterone at varying rates. As a result, suppositories are made with 200 milligrams and 400 milligrams of progesterone.

The minimal doses of progesterone we prescribe for our patients are 200 milligram suppositories for the last eight to sixteen days of the menstrual cycle. Patients with severe cases of PMS who absorb progesterone poorly and metabolize it rapidly may require a 400-milligram suppository four to six times a day for the last ten to eighteen days of the cycle. A patient may need to take the progesterone for six to eight months or for many years. Eventually, for most women, the total dose can be reduced to a minimal amount each day and used only the last four to eight days of the cycle.

Progesterone can be administered orally, intravenously, by injection, in suppositories, or in rectal solution. At some point, it may also be made available in transdermal "patches," nasal spray or drops, or vaginally through slow-release "rings" and artificial membranes, or subcutaneous pellets and microcapsules. At present, the best available means of administering progesterone is the suppository form. Progesterone must be absorbed into the system, raise the blood level of the hormone significantly, and keep it raised to a level sufficient to counteract the symptoms. The suppositories generally do this best. The half-life of progesterone in blood is several minutes, with only a small amount of progesterone stored in body fat. When taken orally, in a pill or liquid, progesterone is rapidly absorbed into the bloodstream and just as rapidly metabolized by the liver to an inactive substance. Consequently, large doses of progesterone would be required for the hormone to be effective by oral administration. But future research may produce an effective oral administration of progesterone.

Intramuscular injectable progesterone reaches a peak blood level within eight hours with the return to base line occuring within eighteen to forty-eight hours. Many women cannot tolerate progesterone injections. When the hormone is suspended in a water base, the injections are extremely painful; when it is suspended in an oil base allergic reactions and sterile abscesses may develop. Nonetheless, progesterone in oil injections should be considered for patients who are hospitalized, where close supervision is required, especially with patients who are suicide risks, or are likely to become involved in child abuse or alcohol abuse, or who show no response to suppositories. If injectable progesterone is required, the starting dose in women who have not had a term pregnancy is 50 mg once or twice daily and in women who have had children, 100 mg once or twice daily. Injections may be supplemented by suppositories or on occasion alternated with suppositories.

Progesterone administered by suppository via the rectum or vagina reaches peak blood level within four to eight hours with the return to base line occurring within twelve to twenty-four hours. Even when the suppositories are absorbed well, a woman may require several administrations per day to maintain adequate blood levels. Some women absorb progesterone poorly via the rectal or vaginal mucosa; a number of factors can affect the absorption rate including the type of base used in the suppository. Women who do not absorb progesterone well may require a suppository that contains more than 200 mg of progesterone, up to a maximum dose of 400 mg per suppository.

A study by Dr. Robert Reid, a Canadian endocrinologist, compared progesterone absorption from three different suppository bases — polyethylene glycol, glycolgelatin, and cocoa butter — demonstrating that peak circulating levels achieved with polyethylene glycol suppositories were significantly higher than either of the other two bases. A polyethylene glycol base or fatty acid base progesterone suppository is available upon prescription by a physician and compounded by pharmacists. Many American pharmacists experienced at compounding are Fellows of the American College of Apothecaries, which is located at 874 Union Avenue, Memphis, Tennessee 38163. The progesterone suppository used safely in England for the past fifteen years has a fatty acid base. No adverse effects have been reported with any of these types of suppositories, although they may cause minor irritation due to mechanical effects. The suppository produced in England may interfere with the effectiveness of vaginal diaphragms used for contraception, according to some reports.

For women who have never been pregnant the starting dosage is 200 to 400 milligrams per suppository daily; for women who have born a child it is 200 to 400 mg twice a day. If after starting progesterone, a woman notices a recurrence of symptoms, she should immediately increase the number of suppositories used each day. Once she increases the number, however, she should not decrease that amount during that particular cycle. If the woman gains no relief after her first course of progesterone, beginning with the next cycle of treatment she should increase the dose of progesterone to 200 mg two or three times a day if she's never had a term pregnancy and up to 400 mg four times a day if she's carried a fetus to term. Higher doses seem to be required by women who have had more pregnancies, and particularly those with a history of toxemia, hypertension in pregnancy, or postpartum depression. A woman who requires more than six 400 mg suppositories per day probably is not absorbing progesterone well and may require the use of a suppository with a different base.

Progesterone is usually administered from the time of ovulation to the onset of menstruation. But timing may need to be adjusted for the following reasons:

1. *Symptoms at ovulation.* Start progesterone two days before expected onset of symptoms.

2. *Irregular and prolonged cycles*. Stop progesterone at time of expected onset of menstruation.

3. *Length of cycle*. Ovulation usually occurs about fourteen days before onset of menstruation except in a short cycle of twenty to twenty-two days when ovulation tends to occur ten to twelve days before the onset of menstruation.

4. *Short episode of symptoms* (lasting only one to five days). Start progesterone three to five days before the expected onset of symptoms.

5. *Symptoms continuing into menstruation*. During the first two to four treatment cycles, discontinue progesterone at the expected onset of menstruation. Often symptoms continuing into menstruation will then cease. If they persist, however, reduce progesterone dosage to one-half the usual dose during the first few days of menstruation, then discontinue.

Once dosage, timing and absorption have been sufficiently achieved and the relief of symptoms has been gained, continue the same dose of progesterone for three symptom-free cycles. Then gradually reduce the dose by starting the course of treatment two days later each month. If the symptoms return, the next month's course should be started at the shortest course producing complete symptom relief and continued for a further two or three symptom-free months before attempting to reduce the dose again. Women in their thirties, especially those who have not had a term pregnancy, often require progesterone therapy for six to twelve months. Women over forty usually need progesterone until menopause. Women between thirty and forty are more difficult to predict in terms of length of treatment. An increasing length of treatment usually is required for women with a number of pregnancies and for those with a history of toxemia or postpartum depression.

Adjustments of Timing

When problems do develop with progesterone therapy, it is usually because the timing of the progesterone treatment needs to be adjusted. Some of the problems with timing and the appropriate adjustments include:

1. *Shortening of cycle*. During the next cycle, start the progesterone one to two days later.

2. *Lengthening of cycle*. Stop progesterone at the time of the expected onset of menstruation, and bleeding will usually occur within 48 hours.

3. *Spotting at mid-cycle* will occur if progesterone is used too early in the follicular phase.

4. *Spotting in the premenstruum*. Stop progesterone, then start the next course of treatment one to two days later.

5. *Erratic cycles*. Usually this is an indication that the patient has forgotten to use her progesterone for one to two days.

6. *Hives or rash*. This may occur as a reaction to the vegetable oil used in injectable progesterone. Discontinue the injections and continue further treatment with suppositories.

The Controversies: The FDA and Cancer

Injectable progesterone in oil is commonly produced in the United States, but progesterone suppositories are not. The suppository form is tolerated best by most women, which is why it is important to make progesterone suppositories readily available throughout the country. Pharmacists are permitted to compound suppositories for individuals upon a physician's prescription. But the research trials necessary to meet Food and Drug Administration regulations must be completed and approved before suppositories can be made by a pharmaceutical manufacturer here.

Obtaining FDA approval for the commercial production and distribution of progesterone depends on the outcome of investigative studies proposed to be carried out at Duke University in cooperation with L.D. Collins Ltd., the British manufacturer of progesterone suppositories, which would like to produce them in this country. Other studies are being carried out by Gail Keith, a nurse practitioner working under the supervision of Dr. W.N. Spellacy at the University of Illnois, at Vanderbilt University Hospital, at the National Institutes of Mental Health, and at our own centers. With the assistance of Dr. Charles Lloyd of Bowman Gray School of Medicine and Dr. Phillip Stubblefield of Massachusetts General Hospital, in 1981 we filed with the F.D.A. the first double-blind, placebo-controlled crossover study sponsored by L.D. Collins Ltd. Unfortunately, the F.D.A. chose to limit that study to a maximum 200 milligram progesterone suppository once a day for the last fourteen days of the cycle. From our clinical experience and that of Dr. Dalton's, we know that this limited dose would be effective in fewew than ten percent of the women with significant PMS. Such a restricted study, we felt, would have been unfair to our patients and a poor use of the limited resources of time, energy, and money. Other academic researchers agreed with us. Subsequently, we withdrew from the study and assisted L.D. Collins in arranging to carry out their studies with the Department of Obstetrics and Gynecology at Duke University, where Dr. Charles Hammond, a prominent gynecologic endocrinologist, is the department chairman. The move to Duke was made with the hope that they could persuade the F.D.A. to allow studies to proceed using higher dosages of progesterone. In early 1983, an advisory committee to the F.D.A. decided after a hearing on the subject that pharmacologic kinetic studies could go ahead. If those studies did not cause greatly elevated blood levels of progesterone, the advisory group said it would approve higher dose clinical studies of progesterone in the treatment of PMS. The results of the pharmacologic kinetic studies were not available as this book was written.

Has progesterone been implicated as a carcinogen? The answer is a resounding no. In fact, progesterone very likely has a cancer preventive quality. A recent study of women evaluated for infertility suggested that a deficiency of progesterone increased the risk of premenopausal breast cancer by 5.4 times and increased the risk of death by all cancer by ten times. That suggests that progesterone is a factor in reducing the incidence of cancer. There's other evidence of progesterone's protective characteristics.

Studies of progesterone's effect on mice, rats, rabbits, and dogs have been similar to research of the progestogens that are used in oral contraceptives.

The progestogens commonly used in oral contraceptives produce tumors in animals. Norethynodrel alone will increase the incidence of pituitary tumors in mice of both sexes and in combination with the estrogen, mestranol, it will increase the incidence of pituitary, vaginal and cervical tumors in female mice and of malignant mammary tumors in rats of both sexes. Ethynodiol diacetate, another progestogen in the Pill, also caused an increased incidence of malignant mammary tumors in female rats. However, we know now that the birth control pill protects women from the risk of some types of cancer. Recent research studies of women who have taken the birth control pill for a significant period of time have demonstrated that oral contraceptives reduce the risk of endometrial cancer by fifty percent and significantly reduce the risk of various disorders, including benign breast disease, ovarian cysts and cancer, pelvic inflammatory disease, iron deficiency anemia, tubal pregnancies, and rheumatoid arthritis.

The research and results of these studies are similar to those for progesterone.

The research studies of progesterone in animals have involved subcutaneous or intramuscular injection of the hormone in mice, rats, rabbits, and dogs, and subcutaneous implantation in mice and rats. Progesterone alone was tested in mice and dogs; in rats it was tested in combination with other chemicals; in mice it was also given in combination with known carcinogens. Given alone it increased the incidence of ovarian, uterine, and mammary tumors in mice. In dogs, long-term, continuous progesterone exposure in high dosages resulted in increases in the incidence of mammary nodules similar to that seen with medroxyprogesterone, a compound related to progesterone. This is viewed as a special circumstance; the results are limited only to experiments with beagles. There is no clinical evidence for a relationship between progesterone use and breast cancer in women. From the experience of the animal research studies with progestogens used in oral contraceptives — which increase the incidence of some tumors in animals but are protective against some tumors in humans — research may well confirm that progesterone is also protective against cancer in humans. In England, where Dr. Katharina Dalton has treated women with premenstrual syndrome for thirty years with progesterone, no in-depth epidemiological study has been undertaken into the long-term effects of progesterone; however, no links between progesterone and incidence of cancer have been reported either. Again, the overall protective effect of progesterone may be illustrated by the sharply reduced cancer risk in women with progesterone deficiencies.

Need for Research

Research studies need to be conducted into progesterone and hormone levels in women with PMS and women without the syndrome. No double-blind control study of progesterone treatment has been done yet despite the hundreds of clinical papers published on related topics. We are preparing just such a study in Massachusetts that will assess the presence of estrogen, progesterone, testosterone, cortex steroid-binding protein, and sex steroid-binding protein in non-PMS and PMS women throughout the cycle. We will see if we can define normal and abnormal estrogen and progesterone hormone ratios, and if it's possible to determine a cut-off point, a point up to which behavior and physical state are normal, and beyond which women experience PMS. These and other investigations will ultimately lead us to discover what causes PMS and why progesterone diminishes the symptoms.

SECTION VII / *The Broader View*

Chapter 27

Fame Is No Protection

The impact of premenstrual syndrome on the behavior of women may explain the erratic, contradictory, or volatile behavior on the part of those who lived before the PMS diagnosis was part of the medical vocabulary. The rich and famous have no immunity to the disorder. We have already seen what appears to have been PMS-like episodes in Lizzie Borden and Joan Crawford. While it is difficult to make precise psycho-historical evaluations without knowledge of a woman's medical history and menstrual cycle, the legacy of biographical material about a number of notable women indicates that premenstrual syndrome may have influenced the behavior of Pauline Bonaparte, Maria Callas, Sylvia Plath, Mary Todd Lincoln, Alice James, and Judy Garland, among others.

Letters, diaries, chronicles and biographies of some members of the British royal family indicate that PMS may have been woven into the fabric of the daily life of Mary Tudor, Katherine of Aragon, Queen Victoria, and perhaps Elizabeth I.

Mary Tudor, the daughter of Henry VIII and Katherine of Aragon, "had not been entirely well since about the age of fourteen, when with the onset of puberty she began to experience symptoms of a disorder known to Renaissance doctors as 'strangulation of the womb' or 'suffocation of the mother,' " writes Carolly Erickson in her book *Bloody Mary*. These terms encompassed various disorders related to the female reproductive system, including amenorrhea, abdominal swelling and bloating, and depression. The range of symptoms that led 16th Century physicians to the diagnosis of strangulation of the womb included headache, nausea, vomiting, lack of appetite, melancholy, and "longing, an ill habit of body, difficulty of breathing, trembling of the heart, swooning, fearful dreams, and watching, with sadness and heaviness." The medical profession then believed that the condition was caused by sexual abstinence. "Every woman, whatever her age, rank or degree of virtue, was at the mercy of her voracious uterus — what for centuries had been called the 'raging womb,' " Erickson writes. Widows, or wives suddenly deprived of the "company of a man," fell into an aggrieved state of melancholy and were troubled with amenorrhea. Even young girls who were strictly kept away from men suffered pain, mental anguish and irregular menstruation, and the only satisfactory cure was marriage. Widows were urged to marry again; wives were advised to engage in "wanton copulation" with their husbands. Physicians told the parents of young girls to arrange matches for them without delay, and in the meantime to send them out horseback riding for several hours a day. No record of the treatments Mary Tudor was given survives, but it is certain that she followed the recommended therapy of daily horseback rides.

Elizabeth Tudor, Queen Elizabeth I, was thought to be healthy, but was known for her periodic, recurring outbursts of virulent temper, Alison Plowden relates in *Elizabeth Regina*. "When stirred to passion, her Highness was quite capable of filling the air with good round oaths and was subject on occasion 'to be vehemently transported with anger.'" Elizabeth in a rage could be heard several rooms away and she was not above throwing things, or boxing the ears of the nearest maid of honor. "When she smiled," wrote her godson, John Harington, "it was a pure sunshine that every one did choose to bask in; but anon came a storm from a sudden gathering of clouds, and the thunder fell, in wondrous manner, on all alike.'"

Victoria's Outbursts

Temper, outbursts, uncontrolled behavior, and the throwing of objects was a pattern laid to Queen Victoria, documented in letters between Prince Albert to the Queen, and in virtually all biographies of her reign. Albert dreaded the outbursts of his wife, primarily because he understood reason better than emotion. Louis Auchincloss in his book *Persons of Consequence, Queen Victoria and Her Circle* writes about these recurring incidents, noting that they may have affected the couple's sex life. "I find it easy to imagine that she may have wanted to make love more frequently than he did, but there is nothing to suggest that he was not usually ready and willing to comply. The Queen was probably fairly easily satisfied; she had no one to compare him with, nobody even to discuss such matters with. Sex must have been an easy price for the peace and quiet that he craved. It may, too, have warded off the temper tantrums that he so dreaded... Outside the bedroom Albert showed, at first, little ability in handling her. When the Queen exploded during arguments and even threw things at him, he would retire to his study to make out a long list of all the reasons that he was right and she was wrong.'' These lists were the famous ''Dear Child'' letters from Albert to Victoria that reveal the cyclical nature of her temper, leading us to conclude that a disorder like premenstrual syndrome may have been the triggering mechanism.

David Duff, in *Albert and Victoria,* writes that the Prince Consort ''knew nothing of the imponderable in women. He was completely inexperienced. He did not appreciate the unreasoned emotions which surged like a maelstrom in Victoria's brain. Albert's answer to all the problems of life was to exercise reason... When Victoria began throwing things and screaming her accusations into his face, he would retire to write a paper on the cause of the outburst... Albert soon learned that any action that he took at such times was wrong. Answering back led to faster, louder vituperation. Remaining quiet was classified as insulting. Retiring behind a locked door eventually led to an attack upon its panels by royal fists. If Albert had taken a stiff whisky, armed himself with a stick and chased Her Majesty along the corridor and up the stairs, he would have discovered that tantrums would have been less frequent and accompanied by less bravado... Even Melbourne, a past master at dealing with women, had on one occasion quavered and feared to sit down as the fire blazed in the eyes of the eighteen-year-old Queen. A cabinet minister was known to fly from her presence, too frightened to follow the rule of withdrawal. (The rule requires those in the Queen's presence to ''back'' out of a room rather than turning about and showing their back to the Queen.) Thus Albert looked forward to the period of pregnancy — it gave emotion a reason... When she was pregnant he was always kind, thoughtful, attentive of her every wish. Here was a problem that he could understand, a train of events to which he could attend.''

Victoria, however, dreaded pregnancy and was disgusted by all things related to menstruation and reproduction. She had difficult pregnancies followed by severe postpartum depression and other complications, again possible evidence of PMS. In *Victoria and the Victorians,* Herbert Tingsten tells us that Victoria ''felt tired and depressed during and after her numerous pregnancies." She also wrote with frankness about marriage. Nuptial night was a shock to her, ignorant as she was in matters of sex. She equated sexual intercourse with the unpleasantness of pregnancy. Looking back on the eve of the wedding of her seventeen-year-old daughter Vicky, Victoria wrote to her: "Yes dearest, it is an awful moment to have to give up one's innocent child to a man, be he ever so kind and good — and to think of all she must go through! I can't say what I suffered, what I felt, what struggles I had to go through — (indeed I have not quite got over it yet) and that last night when we took you to your room, and you cried so much, I said to Papa as we came back 'after all it is like taking a poor lamb to be sacrificed.' You know now — what I meant, dear. I know God has willed it so and that these are the trials which we poor women must go through; no father, no man can feel this! Papa never would enter into it at all! As in fact he seldom can in my very violent feelings."

David Duff also documents these feelings. "Victoria hated being pregnant... She was wearied by the 'constant aches and sufferings, miseries and plagues.' She was bitter at being robbed of her enjoyments, particularly dancing and riding. She felt pinned down, her wings clipped, and only half her real self. She referred to pregnancy as the shadow side of marriage and thought it unfair that men did not take a share of that shadow. A woman, she considered, was morally and physically the man's slave and that, she commented, 'always sticks in my throat... If these selfish men, the cause of all one's misery, only knew what their poor slaves go through.' She thought of herself more in the role of cow than a blessed vehicle giving birth to an immortal soul. The general attitude was not conducive to good temper."

On one occasion, Duff writes, "Queen Victoria and Prince Albert were having tea. Those in attendance upon them noted that Her Majesty had the storm flags flying. There were red patches on her cheeks and her eyes were hard as glass. She raised her cup toward her lips. Then, quick as a flash, she hurled the contents into her husband's face... Before her daughter, the Princess Royal, had been christened, the Queen had become pregnant again. The realization flooded her with depression and anger and she made her feelings very clear to her husband. He, understating as was his habit, informed his brother: 'Victoria is not very happy about it.'"

After the birth of her son, the Prince of Wales, she suffered from severe postnatal depression. She reportedly told King Leopold: "I am very strong as to fatigue and exertion, but not quite right otherwise; I am growing thinner and there is a want of tone... I have likewise been suffering so from lowness that it made me quite miserable, and I know how difficult it is to fight against it."

With our knowledge that a genetic predisposition to PMS exists, it may well be that the syndrome has been a source of medical and psychological problems to current royalty as well.

A Corsican Princess

Another royal princess, Pauline Bonaparte, the sister of Napoleon, may also have suffered from PMS. Pauline is described as a volatile Corsican beauty who shocked European society with her sexual excesses. In *Imperial Venus* by Len Ortzen, we learn that Pauline's first and only pregnancy was a difficult one, whose "effects were to trouble her for many years." She was moody, difficult, had outbursts of temper, and was plagued with medical complaints that made it difficult for her to endure travels by coach and required long hours of rest and the taking of the baths at spas throughout Europe.

"Pauline left the heat of Florence in early July and went at last to Bagni di Lucca," Ortzen writes. "The exact nature of the disorder for which she was seeking a cure is not known; it was not the custom in her day to reveal such details, especially of female ailments, always supposing that they were within the scope of the medical knowledge of the time. Her ailment probably had its origins in the complications following the birth of (her son) Dermide. Her habit of reposing on a chaise-longue, for much longer periods than the prevailing fashion required, and the distress she suffered on long coach journeys, suggest that she was subject to some kind of internal disorder. One of the foremost gynecologists of the day later diagnosed her condition as a chronic inflammation of the womb, accompanied by general prostration and exhaustion."

A letter written by Doctor Jean-Noel Halle, a prominent gynecologist, to her personal physician, Doctor Peyre, discussed this condition. "My dear colleague, I have thought very carefully about the condition of Her Highness and the state of hysteria we found her in yesterday. The womb was still sensitive, though a little less so. The ligaments still exhibited signs of the painful inflammation for which we prescribed baths last Thursday. The spasms in her arms were due to hysteria, as were the pains in her head. Her general state is one of prostration and exhaustion. The inflammation is by no means usual. The present condition of the uterus is caused by a constant and habitual excitation of that organ, and if this does not cease a most grievous condition may result.'' Later, Napoleon's favorite medical adviser Jean-Nicolas Corvisart was summoned from Paris to consult about her health. ''A series of rare complications,'' he wrote, ''has resulted in a condition that is a malady *sui generis,* of which I do not think the exact nature and limits are known. A thousand times unhappy is the Princess who suffers from it, and equally unfortunate are the physicians called in to attend so ambiguous a case.''

Another PMS symptom, increased libido, was experienced by Pauline Bonaparte, who had many love affairs during her marriage to Prince Borghese. One story related by Ortzen is that Pauline ''created a sensation when she commissioned Antonio Canova to carve a statue of her 'almost naked.' He proposed to represent Pauline as Diana the Huntress. But when she learned the legend attached to this goddess, she refused. 'Diana asked her father, Jupiter, to endow her with eternal virginity,' said Pauline. 'If I were represented as that goddess, everyone would have fits of laughter.' It was decided to represent her more appropriately as Venus.''

Mary Todd Lincoln

Abraham Lincoln's wife, Mary Todd Lincoln, has also been portrayed as a woman plagued by recurring, periodic medical and mental disorders that seem to add up to a diagnosis of premenstrual syndrome. Her emotionalism, outbursts, and other complaints, especially migraine headaches and depression, began after the birth of her children — she had four sons. She also had numerous panic attacks and incidents of bizarre behavior. In *Mrs. Abraham Lincoln,* W.A. Evans writes: ''Pregnancy, childbirth, household drudgery, and sick headaches were beginning to tell on this abnormally intense little woman. She was easily frightened into a panic... Mary, finding her child missing, would become hysterical, and, rushing out onto the terrace in front of the house, would scream: 'Bobbie's lost! Bobbie's lost!'... The husband knew, as no one else did, what Mary had to contend with. He had seen her in prostrating, nauseating headaches when her head could not be raised from the pillow and a jarring step on the floor was torture. Lincoln was the only one who knew whether those hysterical outbursts of fear or anger had a time relation to her headaches or to periodic and other ills.'' Abraham Lincoln repeatedly wrote and told friends that ''Mrs. Lincoln is not well.''

After the birth of her fourth child Tad in 1853 she wrote to a friend: ''I have been seriously sick. (My disease is of a womanly nature, which you will understand has been) greatly accelerated by the last three years of mental suffering. Since the birth of my youngest son, for about twelve years, I have been more or less a sufferer.'' Around 1865 an observer noted that ''Mrs. Lincoln's personality included its list of liabilities. In impulsiveness and imprudence, in emotional immaturity, in that tendency to view things personally which shuts out broader wisdom, in susceptibility to flattery, in nervousness aggravated by migraine headaches and the mental tensions of the menopuase, in growing irrationality as to money, she had hidden weaknesses that were to pull her down in one of the most taxing situations a woman ever faced. These defects were not apparent like blindness or a crippled limb. She was like a foot soldier with secret lameness who must march long instances day after day through four years of war. Lincoln at this time was probably finding Mary's moods unpredictable, as has happened to other husbands when their wives reached the forties.'' Another writer noted her periodic, sharp mood swings. ''It was not easy to understand why a lady who could be one day so kindly, so considerate, so generous, so thoughtful and so hopeful, could, upon another day, appear so unreasonable, so irritable, so despondent, so even niggardly, and so prone to see the dark, the wrong side of men and women and events.''

Mary Lincoln's problems grew worse with age, exacerbated by the assassination of her husband and the deaths of three of her sons, and eventually developed into severe depression and other psychiatric disorders that led her at one point to attempt suicide. Eddie Foy, the vaudevillian whose mother was a nurse and companion to Mrs. Lincoln, wrote that she ''had always been a woman of rather unusual disposition.

After her husband's assassination she fell into deep melancholy and after her son Tad died, she suffered from periods of mild insanity. She had many strange delusions.''

Alice James

Alice James, the younger sister of William and Henry James, was another woman whose life was shadowed by periodic recurring illness, anxiety, and psychiatric problems. In her biography of *Alice James,* Jean Strouse paints a picture of a woman so constricted by her health that her life was in many ways very narrow, while intellectually very full. Alice never married, did not bear a child, and produced no great works. From the age of nineteen she was variously described as delicate, fragile, high-strung, nervous, hysterical, and given to prostrations and nervous breakdowns. In many ways, of course, she fulfilled the Victorian ideal of beauty in women, marked, as Strouse notes, by a graceful languor, pallor, and vulnerability. "Illness made a woman ethereal and interesting," observes Strouse. Susan Sontag makes that point in her work, *Illness as Metaphor,* in which she notes that tuberculosis was seen to spiritualize life, a disease almost to be proud of because it was "the sign of a superior nature... a becoming frailty." For Alice James, illness was a part of her life; she was constantly visiting physicians, spas, or sanitariums for the treatment of both physical and mental complaints, although she had periods of good health and enthusiastic, positive mental states as well. But periodically, she suffered episodes of hysteria and paralysis of limbs, suicidal and murderous thoughts. Alice once described wanting to "knock off the head of the benignant pater as he sat with his silver locks, writing at his table," of sitting in the library, reading, when "violent inclinations" made her want to throw herself out the window or harm her father. She wrote of not being able to control her thoughts at school, of "impossible sensations of upheaval" that made it impossible for her to focus and concentrate on her studies. The cycle of good health-ill health is documented by Strouse. At one point she notes, "Since Alice's return from Europe in 1872, her health had gone through its usual (by this time) range of improvements and reversals." In 1878 she had a serious breakdown and became increasingly obsessed with death and suicide. She ultimately developed a tumor, but when she learned of her terminal llness, Strouse says: "Death now seemed to Alice to promise not eternal life but simply peace. It would annihilate all the questions of control, distinction, and selfhood that had plagued her life; it would obliterate the ceaseless conflicts between body and will, male and female, love and hate, good and evil, struggle and acceptance, success and failure. In the face of death, her life took on a new clarity. Death was consummation of struggle and pain, the apotheosis and the cessation of suffering. Alice went out to meet it like a lover keeping a long-awaited assignation, yearning to surrender to its large, dark, over-whelming force."

More Traces of PMS

Premenstrual syndrome may also have been part of the lives of such 20th Century women as Sylvia Plath, Maria Callas, and Judy Garland among others. Judy Garland's volatility, emotionalism, mood swings, depression, insomnia, and many medical problems all worsened after the birth of her three children, notes Christopher Finch in his book, *Rainbow*. She had insomnia in adolescence and mood swings. Her compulsive eating and subsequent weight problem (that had been fairly well controlled during her teens) became a major recurring problem after her pregnancies, which led to her dependence on amphetamines, first used as an appetite suppressant and later, together with alcohol, as a mood-altering substance. Whether her periodic, recurring problems were connected with her menstrual cycle is unclear, but they may well have been.

It is easier to see the cyclical nature of the outbursts, volatility, depression and health problems of opera singer Maria Callas. In her biography *Maria Callas*, Arianna Stassinopoulos details the endless emotionalism and lack of self-esteem of the diva. By examining the dates provided in the biography to many of the incidents, though, we can see a pattern. Almost all of the negative feelings and behavior, health problems, sinus attacks, and binge eating occurred throughout her life from the end of the month through the first ten days — usually from about the 20th to the 10th day. Many happy times and details of Callas' triumphs occurred in the middle of the month. It's a cycle that perhaps could be explained on some other basis, but it fits the pattern of premenstrual syndrome. Callas, according to a friend Francois Valery, had "talked about not feeling good when she had her periods." She suffered from recurring headaches and sinus attacks, as well as violent mood swings. "She became intensely irritable, annoyed by trifles, exaggerating their importance and unable to shake off her excessive concern with them. When she was not irritable she would sulk," Stassinopoulos writes. "Sulks were for Maria a rarely used weapon, but they were a weapon that occasionally took complete control of her... Standing near the pinnacle of worldwide fame, Maria was ambivalent about it, one moment radiant in the attention and admiration and the next moment snappish and resentful in the fear that it would all come to an abrupt end." The episodes are numerous: irritability, rage, grief, losing her voice, problems with her sinuses, emotional quarrels with spouse and manager, fear, shattered nerves, low blood pressure, deep anguish — all of these are variously dated on July 9, December 2, May 31, August 18, January 21, May 29, June 29-30, October 31 by Stassinopoulos. And occasions when the singer was described as in an expansive mood, in peak form, radiant, and feeling fine were dated December 18, August 10, August 15, and so on.

Callas' lack of self-esteem, a natural outgrowth of these cyclical bouts of depression and ill health, was notorious. As Stassinopoulos writes: "Because Maria's store of self-approval remained, most of the time, very low, she came to rely almost entirely on the approval of others. So the woman who had cast her spell on so many was in even greater need of them than they were of her. The greater the adulation the tighter the trap, especially since as she said herself, she was plagued with endless doubt and feelings of unworthiness. 'Even when people look at me with obvious affection, that makes me twice as angry. You think these people are looking at you in admiration — why should they? I don't deserve it.' The less she felt that she deserved admiration, the more she was determined to present to the world a version of herself that was deserving." The frustration and anger that she felt as a result in turn fueled her outbursts and temper tantrums. Depression cloaked the diva for as much as two to three weeks of each month, even when she had much to be happy about. "The end of her year of triumph found Maria in a desperate state. Her dark view of life and the world was once again confirmed, only this time, coming so soon after so much success and so much glory, it was more deeply painful than ever before."

During her prime singing years, we learn she suffered from nervous tension and fueled her performance schedule with food binges, "she was beginning to be increasingly bothered by headaches, fainting spells and attacks of car sickness which she attributed more to the excess weight she carried than to anything else."

Sylvia Plath

Sylvia Plath, whose depression and obsession with suicide were themes woven throughout her poetry and prose, was a woman who clearly had enormous psychiatric problems and suffered with a major clinical depression most of her life. But she may also have had premenstrual syndrome, which could have worsened during a two-year period in which she had two children and a miscarriage and a number of other health problems. Again, by examining the dates of many of her journal entries and examining the material written about her works and the circumstances under which her poetry was written, a pattern seems to emerge. Plath had recurring sinusitis and cyclical mood swings which seem to come and go monthly. The dates of her bad days and good days are very similar to those of Maria Callas — the end and beginning of months seem marked by the worst depressions, suicidal thoughts, and violent feelings while the middle of the months are days of brighter thoughts.

On November 3, 1952, she wrote: "God, if ever I have come close to wanting to commit suicide, it is now, with the groggy sleepless blood dragging through my veins..." On February 18, 1953: "Oh, I would like to get in a car and be driven off into the mountains to a cabin on a wind-howling hill and be raped in a huge lust like a cave woman, fighting, screaming, bitching in a ferocious ecstasy of orgasm... I wonder at my morbid obsession with daydreams." On August 9: "I have never in my life, except that deadly summer of 1953, and fall, gone through such a black lethal two weeks..." On March 28: "Occasionally I lifted my head, ached, felt exhausted. Saturday I groaned, took pellets of Bufferin, stitched in the worst cramps and faintness for months which no pills dulled..." Jan. 22: "Absolutely blind fuming sick. Anger, envy and humiliation. A green seethe of malice through the veins. "But on December 12 she wrote: "Ever since Wednesday, I have been feeling like a 'new person.' Like a shot of brandy went home, a sniff of cocaine, hit me where I live and I am alive and so there." On September 18: "Much happier today — why? Life begins, minutely, to take care of itself — an odd impulse brings a flood of joy, life..." On December 16: "I have been happier this week than for six months." February 10: "How clear and cleansed and happy I feel. Why?"

Clearly, it is impossible to impose explanations on behavior without detailed knowledge of all the influences on feelings, attitudes, and health. But our knowledge of the pervasiveness of premenstrual syndrome in the general female population makes it likely that some of these women whose lives we have studied were influenced to some degree by PMS.

> *"Premenstrual tension is a settled scientific fact, which the law is bound to accept and deal with, just as it must deal with the phenomena of insanity..."*
>
> Howard Oleck, "The Legal Aspects of PMS," 1953.

The Defense Pleads PMS

Between 1970 and 1979 Sandie Craddock, a thirty-year-old English-woman, was convicted of criminal offenses, mostly minor, at least thirty times. She received repeated psychiatric counseling, and her doctors concluded that she suffered a severe personality disorder which led her to seek constant attention. One night in May 1979, she was working in a pub when a dispute broke out, and she stabbed a fellow barmaid to death. While in prison awaiting trial, the monthly pattern of her outbursts was identified as premenstrual syndrome; she was treated with progesterone, and it worked almost immediately. Based largely on the diagnosis of Dr. Katharina Dalton, rather than an independent examination by court-appointed doctors, Craddock was convicted on a lesser charge of manslaughter. The court concluded that her case fit the category of "diminished responsibility," meaning that her medical condition lessened her ability to take responsibility for her actions. The charge was reduced to manslaughter from murder and she was released on three years' probation, with the stipulation that she continue to receive progesterone treatment.

But in the fall of 1980, for reasons that are not made clear in the court record, Craddock went for several days without receiving her usual progesterone treatments. Then, during a trip to a town west of London she tossed a brick through a window. She immediately turned herself in, and was released as soon as her condition and therapy were explained to the local magistrate. In April, 1981, soon after her daily doses were substantially reduced from their initial high levels, Craddock lost control once again. She attempted suicide. In late May she threatened a local police sergeant (whom she accused of being rude to her). Using letters crudely scissored out of newspapers and magazines, she had pasted up the message "I Gona Kill You." Several days later she telephoned the police department and stated that she would kill the sergeant. "I hate him. I'm going to kill him. I'll get him." When she was discovered the next morning outside the police station with an open knife in her jacket pocket, she again threatened the sergeant and was arrested. Sandie Craddock is not the world's most sophisticated criminal, but her case posed some very sophisticated issues for the British legal system. Those questions remain unanswered today and anticipate similar issues that will undoubtedly, in time, confront the American courts.

Historically, defendants have been held responsible for their actions unless they can prove that a disability prevented them from conforming to society's accepted standards of behavior. A central issue is whether the courts should include PMS in that category of diseases which so impair the rational faculties of its victims that they are relieved of responsibility for their actions. Defining those "disabilities" continue to be a point of debate. Insanity is the most accepted of these defenses but in recent years it has come under sharp attack. Critics contend that it is often abused, and that many criminals who pose a continuing danger to society are freed on the basis of questionable expert testimony. Even defenders of the insanity defense, and of its related defenses, concede that it is sometimes misapplied. But they still argue that it would be unjust to hold individuals to a standard of conduct that they are simply unable to meet. So the question for the judicial system becomes: at what point do the courts draw the line between a true disability and lesser conditions that many people must bear as part of everyday life?

Historically, menstrually-related problems were accepted as legal defenses for a range of criminal acts. Three notable cases: Martha Brixey, a servant who without any motive murdered an employer's child in 1845 and made no attempt to avoid detection, was acquitted on the grounds of insanity caused by "obstructed menstruation." Six years later Amelia Snoswell was acquitted of the murder of her infant niece again on the grounds of insanity, this time due to "disordered" menstruation. A woman accused of stealing a fur boa was acquitted in 1845 at Carlisle Quarter Sessions on the grounds of temporary insanity "from suppression of the menses."

Need for Establishment Recognition

Despite the colorful history of the 19th Century, PMS is not widely recognized by the medical or the legal establishment today. Until the medical profession reaches broad agreement that PMS can profoundly influence criminal and violent action, judges are likely to view it with extreme skepticism. "I don't see why it is any different than any other illness," says Alan A. Stone, a professor of law and psychiatry at Harvard Law School and Harvard Medical School, expressing a still common view of the legal profession. "The question is whether such a condition would lead to an inability to substantially conform" to the law, he says. "And I think that is patently absurd." The law will likely not come to grips with PMS until medicine does, and even then it will be an uphill battle.

Even among those who agree that there is overwhelming evidence that PMS causes criminal outbreaks, there remains sharp disagreement about whether it should be permitted as a defense. At one extreme are those who argue that proof of PMS at the time of a criminal action should be sufficient to relieve the woman of all responsibility for her acts. They contend that just as juries are permitted to return a verdict of "not guilty by reason of insanity" because the accused had no control over his actions, women who truly suffer from the disease should be declared not guilty by reason of PMS. Premenstrual syndrome does share some legal characteristics with insanity, but it differs in many key respects.

At the other extreme are those who don't believe that PMS, even if proven to be the motivating factor in a crime, should be permitted as a defense at all. Two distinct groups take this hardline position, but they reach the same conclusion for radically different reasons. One group contends that biology is no excuse for criminal behavior. Males, too, have hormonal imbalances, they point out, but it is impossible to say with certainty how great or little a role those imbalances play in providing a "proximate cause" for criminal behavior.

"Women have long been subject to sexist slurs about hormonal behavior, but modern knowledge is more equanimous," wrote Michael Newman, director of the Warm Spring Harbor Laboratory for Qualitative Biology, in a letter published in The New York Times in 1982. "Male sex offenders, too, have hormonal problems, often high levels of testosterone. And Type A coronary personalities have been found to have very high levels of steroid hormones. It may be that every criminal is chemically deranged. Soon we all may be. The ones who don't hurt people have to be protected from the ones who do.'' What Newman was arguing, in essence, is what lawyers refer to as the ''slippery slope'' problem: allow one type of hormonal imbalance, no matter how severe, to serve as an absolute defense, and soon everyone who claims a similar disorder, no matter how inconsequential, will make a case for special treatment. ''Let the law tamper with small medical knowledge, and what order is left in society will perish with the notion of common sense,'' Newman concluded.

Ardent feminists comprise the second group holding that PMS is no excuse for criminal action. They fear that any legal precedent that establishes women as inferior to men, or brands them with a disability that distorts their ability to think and act logically, may serve as a basis for discrimination. ''It could become a tremendous sword,'' said Elizabeth Holtzman, a former congresswoman who is now District Attorney of Brooklyn, N.Y. ''It could become a basis for refusing to hire women. It could become an excuse to go back to all kinds of discrimination that we have been trying to get away from.''

Others fear that legal recognition of PMS would prompt some to question if a woman with even the slightest symptoms of PMS could be trusted with national security secrets, or could be given the power to launch a nuclear war? Concludes Holtzman: ''I think that we ought to be able to say that women can be held accountable for their acts just as men'' are.

The Middle Course

In between these two extreme views lies a compromise position. That is essentially the stand taken by the British courts in the Craddock case and one other. By declaring that Sandie Craddock suffered from diminished capacity to control her acts, the court was able to enter a verdict of guilty, but reduce her sentence and order proper medical treatment. Logical as the approach seems, diminished capacity is not a formal defense in the United States. Nonetheless, the theory exists, for all practical purposes, in the power of judges to take extraordinary circumstances into consideration when passing sentence. And, with certain safeguards to ensure that the PMS defense is not abused, that is how we believe the American criminal justice system should handle cases involving *bona fide* PMS victims.

In some respects, PMS differs from any diseases, both of the mind and the body, that have previously confronted the judicial system. The cyclical nature of PMS episodes defies most legal categories. Temporary insanity and other mental disorders occur in fits and starts, not in cycles. A PMS victim, however, may be perfectly normal for all but a few days, sometimes a week or two, each month. Because her violent actions are likely to recur regularly, they cannot be dismissed by a judge as a singular event unlikely to repeat itself. At the same time, her acts cannot be regarded as symptomatic of a permanent condition that requires institutionalization for the protection of society and the patient.

The premise of Western law is that citizens are held responsible for their actions when they are in control of their rational faculties. When they are not, judges and juries have an added responsibility to ensure that the criminal receives treatment, not punishment. At the same time, they still have a responsibility to ensure that the community is protected against violent acts, whether rationally motivated or not. For 150 years, lawyers and lawmakers have argued over how to define the law so that both responsibilities are met. They are still arguing. As we have seen, the complications of a PMS case have not yet reached a United States court. But they have been anticipated in a number of scholarly journals and law review articles, the most articulate and thorough of which is a comprehensive study published in 1971 in the *Law Review of the University of California, Los Angeles*. The authors, Aleta Wallach and Larry Rubin, concluded that PMS victims must be "assured the same medical and legal rights purportedly accorded to those who suffer from similar defects and diseases." But they admitted, and later writings have confirmed, that nothing is similar enough to resolve the thorny legal questions.

What has become clear is that PMS falls into a legal no-man's land between insanity and "automatism," the condition in which an individual acts automatically and without conscious knowledge of his acts. As a result, when faced with PMS cases, judges are likely to rely heavily on insanity, automatism, and other instances in which organic or biological events play a decisive role in patterns of behavior. Insanity, the best known and most controversial of the defenses, is a good starting point. Both the American and British definitions of insanity harken back to the case of Daniel M'Naughton, who was accused of killing a member of Parliament in 1843. In M'Naughton's case, it was established that one can use insanity as a defense if "the party accused was laboring under such a defect of reason, from disease of the mind, as not to know the nature and quality of the act he was doing; or, if he did it, that he did not know he was doing what was wrong."

PMS, like some other diseases that have brought the M'Naughton rule under criticism, does not quite fit the bill. First, it is not at all clear that PMS is a "disease of the mind," as we have illustrated throughout this book. Secondly, there is no evidence that PMS victims, even while in the most violent fits, are unaware of their actions, or do not know that the actions are wrong. In that regard, the disease resembles kleptomania, pyromania, and other conditions in which the criminal action is the result of an "irresistible impulse." Some states have broadened the M'Naughton rule, making the insanity defense available to those who are unable to control their actions even if they fully understood their implications. Under this definition, PMS and insanity, or at least temporary insanity, bear a close resemblance.

The problem with allowing an "irresistible impulse" as a defense, however, is that some illnesses seem to involve not only "impulses" but careful planning and premeditation. (Sandie Craddock, it should be remembered, talked about her attempted murder of the sergeant over a period of several days.) In 1954, in *Durham v. United States*, the U.S. Court of Appeals tried to avoid this distinction with the simpler, if broader statement that "an accused is not criminally responsible if his unlawful act was the product of mental disease or mental defect." Predictably, the effort at simplification only added more complications. First, it treated the mind as a separate entity, divorced from the body's biological activities. Secondly, the Durham rule made it necessary to prove that the act was the "product" of the defect, a nearly impossible standard to meet with one hundred percent certainty.

Still a third test, devised by the American Law Institute, says that there should be no responsibility for criminal conduct if the accused "lacks substantial capacity either to appreciate the criminality of his conduct or to conform his conduct to the requirements of the law." That eliminates some of the ambiguity of the Durham rule, but it is of little help in figuring out how to treat PMS victims. Except when they endure periodic episodes, they know as well as any citizen the difference between right and wrong. And even when controlled by strong impulses, they usually know if they are doing something they should not be doing.

In short, insanity differs too much from PMS to be of any real help in fashioning legal guidelines. Broadly speaking, under almost any insanity test, a defendant must show that her mental state prevented her from premeditating, deliberating, entertaining malice toward her victim, or holding the intent to kill. At various times, a PMS victim might demonstrate all of these characteristics.

In some ways, PMS should pose fewer difficulties for the courts than insanity. The cyclical behavior of PMS victims make it easier to determine who has the disease and who is faking it. The symptoms, while varying from individual to individual, are not as variable as those of insanity. More importantly, even if PMS victims could be treated like the the insane in the eyes of the law, it would not likely be in their best interest to be so. A successful insanity plea means that the court is free to institutionalize the defendant for an indefinite time period. With an illness like PMS, in which effective therapy with progesterone can control the symptoms, there is no evidence that incarceration would do anything but isolate the victim from society. It would have no "reforming" effect. Moreover, it would equate women who suffer from PMS with those who our society has said must be wards of the state because they cannot function on their own.

The law has not only relieved the insane from responsibility for their actions; it has, in some cases, found that the non-insane may also be subject to "irresistible impulse." The case law in this area has been inconsistent, and it has embraced a wide range of abnormalities. But most common among the "non-insane" defenses is automatism, an altered state of consciousness during which one's personality changes suddenly, but usually in a limited way. Usually automatism is accompanied by amnesia, or selective amnesia. Often it is triggered by a traumatic event, such as rejection by a lover. The defense has been used to explain murders, assaults, and attempts to evade the police, among other events.

The first problem raised by such claims is proof. In most countries, the courts have ruled that it is not enough simply to claim automatism; some evidence must sustain the contention. Thus, there is almost no way to sustain the automatism defense of someone who committed an unwitnessed crime. But a man named Gottschalk, accused of theft and assault in Canada in 1975, was acquitted primarily because witnesses who saw him immediately after the crimes said that he appeared to be in a state of shock. That testimony corresponded with the findings of a psychiatrist who examined the defendant. The Gottschalk decision and others like it have been criticized because the acquittal set the defendant free without any requirement that he obtain treatment — an unlikely result had he been found not guilty by reason of insanity. There is no assurance that his "non-insane" condition will not return. Indeed, the line between automatism and temporary insanity is a thin one, and it is unclear where one condition begins and the other ends.

Similar defenses have been offered by those who suffer from "post traumatic stress disorder," which has also been called "Vietnam syndrome," because it is commonly found among veterans who have survived heavy combat. They suffer a delayed reaction to the immense stress of the front lines. The symptoms resemble those of automatism: often a recurring sound or sight, like helicopter noise, brings on a dissociative state. It is a temporary condition. The syndrome was used successfully as a defense in the case of a Vietnam veteran who held a guard captive at a congressman's district office in California. Another received a suspended sentence after pleading that the stress disorder led him to take a church congregation hostage one Sunday afternoon.

Both automatism and post-traumatic stress disorder have been much criticized as legal defenses because they rely so heavily on expert psychiatric testimony. Usually the defendants seek to prove that the disorder was a one-time occurrence, explained by some unusual aspect of their personal history or medical background. Both differ from insanity in that they are singular events, usually prompted by an external stimulus. In many cases, though, the line between these afflictions and temporary insanity is a blurry one. It is extraordinarily difficult to make the distinction, and that explains the inconsistency of the verdicts. But in many cases juries have been convinced that a cause-and-effect relationship exists between the disorder and the criminal action.

Documentation Possible

Critics of the insanity defense, whose ranks have grown since the acquittal of John Hinkley, the attempted assassin of President Reagan, say that such defenses open a Pandora's box. They may be right. More often than not, at least one medical expert can be found to back every contention, however frivolous. Could the same criticism be made of the PMS defense? Yes, especially if it is diagnosed by "experts" who are simply hired hands aiding the execution of legal legerdemain. But extensive psychiatric testimony is not necessary to prove the existence of PMS, as it is for insanity, automatism, and post-traumatic stress disorder. The cyclical nature of PMS lends itself to careful documentation that should establish beyond any doubt whether the defendant truly suffers from the disease, or whether she is simply using it.

Dr. Estelle Ramey, a professor of physiology and biophysics at the Georgetown University Medical School, is also a researcher into the effects of sex hormones. She says that PMS has a place in the courtroom "if you can establish that a woman in her past history belongs to the group of women who are really disabled, emotionally and physically, during this period." Dr. Dalton suggests that the plea of PMS requires a woman to "produce positive evidence of similar episodes of loss of control, confusion, amnesia or violence" in the three previous menstrual cycles. Such evidence, she says, might be supplied by the woman's employer, friends or family, or by searching through diaries, medical files, police records, or prison documents. Moreover, the characteristics of the crime should very nearly match the typical profile of the PMS sufferer: she should have been acting alone, the event should not have been premeditated (usually; there are exceptions), the action should have occurred without a clear motive, there should be almost no attempt to escape detection. Imposing such a stiff standard is the only way to ensure that the PMS defense is not diluted by constant use and abuse. Dalton applauds the rejection of the PMS plea made by a travel agent's clerk accused of absconding with travelers' checks. The defendant said she suffered from PMS, but could only narrow the date of the crime to a nine-month period.

A highly publicized case in Brooklyn, N.Y. in 1982 that promised to be the first litigated case of the PMS defense in the United States was similarly ill-starred. A Legal Aid attorney representing Shirley Santos, a twenty-five-year-old mother of six accused of child abuse, announced her intention to use PMS as the defense because the defendant had said the incident occurred on the first day of her period. The District Attorney of Brooklyn is Elizabeth Holtzman, a former congresswoman who is a feminist and champion of women's rights; she has also adopted a conservative view of her role as prosecutor and keeps herself and her cases very much in the public eye. Legal Aid vs. Holtzman drew enormous pre-hearing publicity and promised to be a precedent-setter for the PMS defense in this country. Holtzman clearly was not going to move from her position, repeated in interview after interview, on *The Phil Donahue Show,* with *The New York Times* and in half a dozen press conferences. "I have long argued that there is no basis for the use of this defense," she told *The New York Times.* "There is no scientific evidence that there is any such thing as a syndrome which causes women to become insane or violent in connection with the menstrual cycle."

Behind the publicity and press conferences, the case itself was springing leaks. The harm to the child was minor, which made the case ripe for plea-bargaining. No information indicating that Shirley Santos had premenstrual syndrome, or had ever experienced PMS-type episodes in previous menstrual cycles, or had ever been treated for recurring cyclical health problems apparently existed. It was a bad case at the wrong time to start with, but it was torpedoed by the defendant herself. Shirley Santos, interviewed on local television at the courthouse when a scheduled hearing was postponed, looked right into the camera and said that PMS: "isn't my defense, it's my lawyer's... My nerves are not that bad that I am just going to beat up on my kid because my period comes down." Compounding the problems was a sudden strike by Legal Aid attorneys, which caused one postponement of the Santos hearing, and, legal observers in the Brooklyn court district said, contributed to the mutual decision to settle the case out of court. Appearing before Judge Donald Jacobi on November 3, 1982, Santos said she struck her daughter, Quadina, when she refused to be quiet. Pleading guilty to a lesser charge of harassment, which is a violation not a crime, she was given a conditional discharge with the stipulation that she would continue for a year in a counseling program. At a news conference afterward, Holtzman said, "The withdrawal of this defense is a signal that PMS is a defense without merit." The District Attorney conceded that many women experience "irritability, depression, and pain accompanying the menstrual cycle," but nothing constituting a condition that would justify a legal defense. In any event, she added, Santos had undermined any claim to such a defense when she disavowed the syndrome in the memorable television interview.

In a letter to *The New York Times* published November 15, Stephanie Benson, the Legal Aid attorney for Santos, "respectfully" disagreed. "I wholeheartedly believe that without the PMS arguments Miss Santos would still be facing criminal charges. The fact that they were all dropped is, instead, a testament to its validity... My hope is that in the future women with such difficulties will be able to recognize and receive appropriate treatment for them — free of social stigma or ill-conceived fear of economic reprisals."

Given the predominance of premenstrual syndrome in the population at large, it is only a matter of time before a woman, somewhere, sometime, finds herself swept up in an incident that she didn't plan, didn't intend, wouldn't have conceived of doing, outside of a premenstrual episode. When that happens, the American judicial system will be confronted with the PMS defense. Until an actual courtroom drama unfolds, we can only speculate about the issues and responses.

Our courts would do well to borrow from the British concept of diminished responsibility, which in the words of one legal scholar would allow the jury "to mitigate the punishment of a mentally disabled but sane offender in any case where the jury believes that the defendant is less culpable than his normal counterpart who commits the same criminal act." The criminal act is judged by the standards of the community — standards that a PMS sufferer, during much of the month, can appreciate, understand, and obey. At the same time, the sentence would reflect the extenuating circumstances under which the crime was committed. This approach does not preclude a jail term, especially for repeat offenders. But it makes proper medical treatment a likelihood. It is a practical approach. The issue of guilt or innocence can be decided without reference to the disease, an approach that should be more satisfactory both to feminists and those concerned that every hormonal imbalance may soon be offered as a defense. And until the existence of PMS is widely recognized, judges will likely be more amenable to adopting a system over which they have more personal control.

An exemplary case in this regard occurred in England only a few months after the Craddock case. In December 1980, thirty-seven-year-old Christine English, a woman with a long history of treatment for depression and premenstrual syndrome, had a series of raging, no-holds-barred battles with the man whom she was seeing regularly; he was married, an alcoholic, and an inveterate philanderer. On the night in question he planned to meet another woman. Christine English picked him up at a pub, where he had gotten drunk, and apparently agreed to drive him around in search of the woman he was supposed to meet. During the drive, they resumed their fight; he got out of the car. She drove away. But suddenly she made a U-turn, accelerated and drove the car directly at him, pinning him to a streetlamp. He died days later. Under the Homicide Act of 1957, English's history of PMS enabled her to plead guilty to a reduced charge of manslaughter. The judge heard testimony indicating that at the time of the murder she was in a state of great hormonal imbalance. Instead of sentencing her to prison, the judge put her on probation, ordered her to receive treatment — and forbade her to drive a car.

Both the Craddock and English decisions drew headlines and news reports in Britain and around the world. Fleet Street journalists made much of the implications of murder without punishment. But serious journals repeated the basic questions posed by PMS: "Despite legal cases which seem to have established the premenstrual syndrome as a mitigating condition in women who commit serious crimes, the disease status of the syndrome is seriously questioned," opined *The Lancet*. An article in *New Society*, "*Do Women Go Mad Every Month?*" concluded that accepting PMS as a mitigating factor in murder cases was not likely to serve the interests of women. What these and other critics neglect to consider is that a small number of women have been observed to have a severe and extreme disorder that occasionally causes them to do things in an uncontrollable state that they would not consider doing when they are symptom-free. Few of them are criminals, with intention and motive; little purpose would be served by incarcerating women whose only crime is a physiological defect beyond their control. What they do need is treatment. That was the basis of the sentences in the Craddock and English cases, which balanced the demands of society to protect itself from and punish criminals, with the more fundamental need to rehabilitate and make whole a transgressor. When progesterone therapy can "rehabilitate" a woman with PMS, why should she be imprisoned at great cost to the taxpayer in an environment that can breed crime rather than eradicate it? The aim of the law, after all, is to protect society and to aid and reform the individual. The magistrates in the English and Craddock cases bore the aim in mind, and recognized and ordered treatment for the disease.

Chapter 29

"We should all be concerned about the future because we will have to spend the rest of our lives there."

Charles Franklin Kettering, Seed for Thought

Making Progress

"To me, PMS is a woman's issue," one of our patients says. "It's equal health. Equal pay and equal jobs aren't going to do women any good if they're not well enough to take them." We agree, but not everyone does. The outcry over premenstrual syndrome that was triggered by the attempted use of the disorder as a legal defense is likely to expand by geometric progressions as information about PMS travels. Some feminists have already staked out the battlefield, charging that an acceptance of PMS is a tacit assumption that women are biologically disadvantaged, incapable of rational decision-making because of their vulnerability to monthly hormonal surges. They fear its recognition will lead to a regression, taking us backward to a pre-liberation world in which women are denied responsible jobs, promotions, political victories, and academic appointments because of their hormonal fluctuations.

The Feminist Debate

The feminist tendency to batten down the hatches, foreclosing attacks on women's abilities, is more understandable in light of the notoriety of certain sexist arguments. It was Dr. Edgar Berman who exploited the term "raging hormones" in a 1970 debate with Dr. Estelle Ramey, the Georgetown University Medical School professor. "Men and women are programmed more than we ever thought we would be," he says. "It's all evolutionary and genetic... Just as the rowdy kiddies of the 60s went back to home economics and dental school at the birth of the 70s, so shall this feminist uprising recede into history in the 80s." His view: "I just don't think you can make a Doberman pinscher out of a French poodle, or a Nelson Bunker Hunt out of a Bo Derek." Last year Berman renewed the furor over the biological differences between men and women in a polemic *The Compleat Male Chauvinist*.

Even the feminists aren't denying the biological differences between men and women but they are concerned about how these differences are perceived by society as a whole and used by women themselves. Susan Brownmiller, author of *Against Our Will*, takes a more measured view of PMS than some, but is extremely critical of its role as a legal defense. Brownmiller told us in an interview, "There are tremendous biological differences. But biological differences are not an excuse for violent crime." She calls a PMS legal defense "special case pleading" by women. "It's falling on the mercy of the court because you are a woman. Are men going to plead that it is an excess of testosterone that drives them to crime? I don't believe that PMS could drive a woman to a criminal act, unless she had crime on her mind... We are rational people who know what a violent crime is." Brownmiller continues, "I do not support it as a legal defense. As a legal defense it is very dangerous. It's not an excuse for a crime." She does not accept a defense that "relieves you of the responsibility of your actions... unless you're totally crazy," she says, which indicates she has some acceptance of the insanity defense.

Yet Brownmiller concedes that premenstrual syndrome exists as a disorder affecting many women. "I *know* it exists... As far as irritability or bursting into tears, I can see it for that." She told us in an interview that she feels that PMS "is neither positive or negative" in terms of a woman's issue. "It's something that should be dealt with."

Liz Creighton, who owns an engineering company in California, was among the women reluctant to recognize the existence of premenstrual syndrome. "I didn't really want to think I was subject to raging hormones." But since progesterone therapy has worked so effectively for her, she says it's better to accept the problem "and bring it out of the closet." What changed her attitude, she says flatly, "was being treated. Realizing that it was a problem that could be treated. I was ready to try anything. It was a question of my life." A major part of her problem in dealing with PMS, she recalls, was her deep-felt insistence on not being burdened by "women's problems... My generation was not going to be burdened with 'the curse,' As soon as I started menstruating I decided that it wasn't going to stop me; I was going to swim, wear Tampax, live a life. This denial started very early on." She says her mother in a way contributed to the denial: "She saw to it [by telling her about menstruation] that I wasn't going to go through the trauma she went through." She takes issue with Brownmiller's rigid denial that the PMS disorder can lead to a loss a control. "When I wasn't suffering from PMS, I *could* control myself. My anger was uncontrollable [during PMS]. It was hurting my work. I was getting more and more ineffective. I was reluctant to take on new projects because I was no longer sure if I would be able to handle them. It brought on a crisis of confidence."

Eliminating the Stigma

There should be no stigma attached to a woman who has a physiological disorder. And that is precisely what PMS is. We feel that the real feminist issue is the abysmal disregard of women by the male-dominated medical community, the years of misdiagnosis and improper or lack of treatment for the condition. By acknowledging the existence of PMS and moving quickly to treat it properly, discrimination against women with PMS will end. To do this, we first must go public with the facts about the condition and stop attaching labels like "raging hormones" to women with PMS. As Creighton says, "This was never an easy trauma for me to talk about. Of course, it's easier now, because I'd like to see other women get help. If we hide it, and don't bring it out and get help, we really are limiting ourselves." I think the women who are seeking treatment now "are women like me. They are aggressive and intelligent enough to feel that they deserve control over their own bodies." While some of her women friends and physicians have not been supportive of her PMS-related problems, Creighton says, "Men I know and work with know other women who have PMS. They try to get them to get help. The men see the problem recurring cyclically and are more apt to make the first diagnosis."

The balancing act surrounding PMS — the need to protect women from external attacks from those who would label them as hormonally inferior and the necessity of responding to their internal physical disorder — will ultimately serve to resolve the controversy about the syndrome. For once the physiological condition is properly treated and the symptoms are eliminated, there will be no phases of "raging hormones" or periods of erratic behavior for anyone to cite as evidence of women's biological weakness.

Need for Education

No current medical school textbook — on obstetrics-gynecology, psychiatry, or general medicine — provides more than a paragraph of information on premenstrual syndrome. While some university medical schools have begun to offer an occasional special lecture on the subject, PMS is not part of the curriculum and physicians-to-be are not held responsible for learning about its symptoms and treatment. Before a doctor can diagnose a condition he has to be taught that it exists, what its symptoms are and what the best therapy is. Not only must medical schools integrate material about PMS into their curricula but continuing education seminars and publications must be made available to practicing physicians, not only in America but around the world. The incidence of premenstrual syndrome surpasses that of lung cancer, diabetes, and arthritis in women; that's a reality to which the medical profession must respond.

As we have explained in the course of this book, many women with premenstrual syndrome are chronically ill. Their symptoms recur cyclically over long periods of time and lead them to seek advice and treatment from many different specialists at different times. Premenstrual syndrome alone probably accounts for a very hefty percentage of the health-care visits of women between the ages of eighteen and forty-four, the group that accounts for the largest number of female visits to physicians. Not only are women with PMS among the most aggressive and vocal consumers of health care in this country but they are also the most disenchanted. As a patient of ours who suffered with PMS for fifteen years before receiving appropriate treatment said: "When you go to the best endocrinologist in town and she or he can't do anything for you, and you traipse from doctor to doctor for years, you lose total faith in the medical profession.

As information and education about PMS is circulated and more physicians begin to treat the disorder, women will benefit as well as society. This should also ease demands on the health-care delivery system and improve its efficiency, by eliminating hundreds of thousands of physician and hospital visits each year that had been made by women who were repeatedly misdiagnosed or mistreated for symptoms that were actually manifestations of PMS. And it should also lower health-care costs for many women, who will be able to obtain evaluation and treatment quickly instead of spending months and years in repeated visits to various specialists for PMS symptoms.

Filling the Emotional Needs

Providing emotional and psychological support for the women and their families is another important kind of treatment. Two national nonprofit organizations founded by women with PMS — the National PMS Society and PMS Action — have taken giant steps toward filling this need by organizing local support groups in communities around the country where women can meet and share with other PMS sufferers their experiences. The National PMS Society, founded in 1981 by Lindsey Leckie and Patty Cannon, has set up affiliated support groups in many communities around the country. PMS Action, founded in 1980 by Virginia Cassara with the assistance of Julie Egger, provides information and counseling about PMS; with the help of Beth Jones, PMS Action also presents seminars about the disorder. Both groups help women find physicians in their area who treat PMS. Cassara herself has PMS; after a futile four-year search for medical treatment in this country, she finally traveled to London for evaluation and treatment by Dr. Katharina Dalton in the late 1970s. Upon her return, she began to disseminate information about PMS and progesterone therapy.

More and better research into PMS is also critical. So far the diagnosis and treatment of premenstrual syndrome has been based on the limited investigations of a few dedicated pioneers, notably Dr. Katharina Dalton. But no one has invested the time, money, and effort to undertake directed research — the double-blind controlled studies — that must be done to uncover the cause of the disorder and to answer a score of questions: whether PMS is one or several disorders, what are its causes, what role sex hormones play in the illness, how progesterone acts to alleviate the symptoms, what the long-term effects of progesterone therapy are, whether other therapies might be effective or more effective as a treatment, whether PMS is hereditary, whether progesterone is protective against cancer. To this end, we are undertaking a number of research studies that should begin to provide the answers to these questions. Other researchers at universities in this country, in Canada and Europe have also begun sex hormone research that is likely to broaden our understanding of premenstrual syndrome.

Now that PMS has come out of the closet and attention has begun to be focused upon it, women can look forward to the day when premenstrual syndrome can be treated readily and effectively.

For information about support groups in your area, contact:

The National PMS Society
P.O. Box 11467
Durham, N.C. 27703

PMS Action
P.O. Box 9326
Madison, Wisconsin 53715
(608) 274-6688

For more information about premenstrual syndrome, its evaluation and treatment, contact:

PMS Program Inc.
800 Eastowne Drive
Chapel Hill, N.C. 27514
or
PMS Program Inc.
40 Salem Street
Lynnfield, Mass. 01940

For information about the non-profit, tax-exempt foundation to support research into premenstrual syndrome and develop educational programs for health-care professionals, or to make a tax-exempt contribution, write:

National PMS Foundation Inc.
P.O. Box 3798
Portland, Oregon 97208-3798

Chapter Notes

Chapter 1 PMS: What It Is and What It Isn't

Robert T. Frank. "Hormonal Causes of Premenstrual Tension." *Archives of Neurology and Psychiatry*, 26: 1053, 1931.

Paula Weideger. *Menstruation and Menopause*. New York: Alfred A. Knopf, 1976, pp. 135-137.

Helene Deutsch. *The Psychology of Women*. New York: Grune and Stratton, 1944, vol. I, pp. 166-167.

K. Jean and R. John Lennane. "Alleged Psychogenic Disorders in Women—A Possible Manifestation." *New England Journal of Medicine*, 288, February, 1973.

Sheila MacLeod. *The Art of Starvation*. New York: Schocken Books, 1982, p. 4.

Lawrence Sanders. *The Third Deadly Sin*. New York: Berkley Books, 1982.

Brian Moore. *I Am Mary Dunne*. New York: The Viking Press, 1966.

Estelle Ramey. "Men's Cycles (They Have Them Too, You Know)." *Ms.* 8-14, Spring, 1972.

Telephone interview, Dr. William Keye, assistant professor of obstetrics and gynecology, University of Utah Medical Center, Salt Lake City.

Telephone interview, Brian Moore, Toronto, Canada.

Katharina Dalton. "A Guide to Premenstrual Syndrome and Its Treatment." K. Dalton, London, 1981.

Chapter 2 Eve's Curse

Pliny the Elder. *Natural History*, Book 7, translated by H. Rackham. Cambridge, Mass.: Harvard University Press, 1961.

Soranus. *Gynecology*, translated by Owsei Temkin. Baltimore: Johns Hopkins University Press, 1956.

Margaret Mead. *Male and Female*, New York: Dell Publishing Company, 1970.

Ruth Benedict. *Patterns of Culture*. Boston: Houghton Mifflin, 1934.

Mary Chadwick. *Psychology of Menstruation*, New York and Washington: Nervous and Mental Disease Publishing Company, 1932.

O.W. Smith and G. van S. Smith. "Menstrual Toxin," in Menstruation and Its Disorders, E.T. Engle ed. Springfield, Ill.: Charles C Thomas Publisher, 1950.

Alison Kane and Eric T. Carlson. "A Different Drummer: Robert B Carter and Nineteenth Century Hysteria." *Bulletin of the New York Academy of Medicine*, 58,6: 519-529, September 1982.

Sigmund Freud. *Totem and Taboo*, Harmondsworth, Middlesex: Penguin Books, 1938.

Raymond Crawfurd. "Superstitions of Menstruation." *The Lancet* December 18, 1915.

Sheila MacLeod. *The Art of Starvation*, op. cit., pp. 38-40.

Erik Erikson. *Identity Youth and Crisis*. New York and London: W.W. Norton and Company, 1968.

Vern Bullough and Martha Voght. "Women, Menstruation, and Nineteenth-Century Medicine." *Bulletin of Historical Medicine*, 47: 66-82, 1973.

British Medical Journal, Letters, 1878

Maudsley. *Sex in Mind and in Education*. New York: James Miller, 1884.

S. Icard. *La Femme Pendant la Periode Menstruelle*. Paris: Felix Alcan, 1890, p.136.

Mary Jacobi. *The Question of Rest for Women During Menstruation*, 1876.

Leta Hollingworth. *Functional Periodicity: An Experimental Study of the Mental and Motor Abilities of Women During Menstruation*. New York: Teachers College, 1914.

For an overview of the cultural and social attitudes toward menstruating women and the taboos surrounding menstruation, the following provide basic references:

Sir James Frazer. *The New Golden Bough*, London: S.G. Phillips Inc., 1959.

Bruno Bettelheim. *Symbolic Wounds*. New York: Collier Books, 1962.

Janice Delaney, Mary Jane Lupton and Emily Toth. *The Curse, A Cultural History of Menstruation*, New York: E.P. Dutton & Co., 1976.

Simone deBeauvoir. *The Second Sex*. New York: Alfred A. Knopf, 1952.

Mary Douglas. *Purity and Danger: An Analysis of Concepts of Pollution and Taboo*. Baltimore: Penguin Books, 1970.

Barbara Ehrenreich and Deirdre English. *Complaints and Disorders, The Sexual Politics of Sickness*. Old Westbury, N.Y.: The Feminist Press, 1973.

The following medical papers are cited in order of their appearance in the text:

Robert T. Frank. *The Female Sex Hormone*. Springfield, Illinois and Baltimore: C.T. Thomas, 1929.

Robert T. Frank. "The Hormonal Causes of Premenstrual Tension," *Archives of Neurology and Psychiatry*, New York, 1931.

Alexandre Jacques Francois Brierre de Boismont. "De la menstruation, consideree dans ses rapports physiologiques et pathologiques." Paris: Germer-Bailliere, 1842.

Senator New York: W. Wood and Company, 1878.

Icard. op. cit.

J.D. Morgan. "Menstrual Arthritis." *American Journal of Obstetrics*, New York, 1907, Ivi: 207-210, pp. 235-238.

M.E. Binet. "Crises Gastriques Premenstruelles et Lithiase Biliare." *Tribune Medicale*, Paris, 1909, XLI, 133-136.

Ruth Okey and Elda I. Robb. "Studies of the Metabolism of Women. Variations in the fasting Blood Sugar Level and in SUgar Tolerance in Relation to the Menstrual Cycle." *Journal of Biological Chemistry,* 65: 165-189, 1925.

Robert T. Frank. "Clinical Data Obtained with the Female Sex Hormone Blood Test," *Journal of the American Medical Association,* January 14, 1928.

W.A. Thomas. "Generalized Edema Occurring Only at Menstrual Period." *Journal of the American Medical Association,* 101: 1126-1127, October 7, 1933.

J.S. Sweeney. "Menstrual Edema; preliminary report." *Journal of the American Medical Association,* 103: 234-236, July 28, 1934.

A.J. Ziserman. "Ulcerative Vulvitis and Stomatitis of Endocrine Origin." *Journal of the American Medical Association,* 104: 826, March 9, 1935.

S. L. Israel. "Premenstrual Tension." *Journal of the American Medical Association,* 110: 1721-1723, May 21, 1938.

E.C. Hamblen. *Endocrine Gynecology.* Springfield, Illinois: C.C. Thomas, 1939.

J. Geber. "Desensitization in the Treatment of Menstrual Intoxication and Other Allergic Symptoms", *British Journal of Dermatology,* 51: 265-268, June 1939.

J.P. Greenhill and S.C. Freed. "Mechanism and Treatment of Premenstrual Distress with Ammonium Chloride." *Endocrinology,* 26: 529-531, March 1940.

L. A. Gray. "The Use of Progesterone in Nervous Tension States." *Southern Medical Journal,* 1004-1010, September 1941.

Morton S. Biskind. "Nutritional Deficiency in the Etiology of Menorrhagia, Metrrohagia, Cystic Mastilis and Premenstrual Tension, Treatment with Vitamin B Complex." *Journal of Clinical Endocrinology and Metabolism,* 3: 227-234, 1943.

Benjamin N. Tager and Shelton Kost. "Personality Changes in Endocrine Disorders." *Journal of Clinical Endocrinology and Metabolism,* 239-242, 1943.

Harvey E. Billig Jr. and S. Charles Spaulding Jr. "Hyperinsulinism of Menses." *Industrial Medicine,* 16: 336-339, July 1947.

Stieglitz and Kimble. "Premenstrual Intoxication," *American Journal of Medical Sciences,* 1949.

E.Y. Williams and L.R. Weekes. "Premenstrual Tension Associated with Psychotic Episodes," *Journal of Nervous and Mental Diseases,* 116: 321-329, 1952.

W. Bickers. "Premenstrual Tension and its Relationship to Water Metabolism." *American Journal of Obstetrics and Gynecology,* 64: 587-590, September 1952.

Joseph H. Morton. "Premenstrual Tension," *American Journal of Obstetrics and Gynecology,* 60: 343-352, 1950.

R.E. Hemphill. "Incidence and Nature of Puerperal Psychiatric Illness." *British Medical Journal,* 2: 1232-1235, December 6, 1952.

Katharina Dalton and Raymond Green. "The Premenstrual Syndrome," *British Medical Journal,* May, 1953.

British Medical Journal, Editorial, 1953.

Linford Rees. "Psychosomatic Aspects of the Premenstrual Tension Syndrome," *Journal of Mental Sciences,* 62-73, January 1953.

Harvey E. Billig Jr. "The Role of the Premenstrual Tension in Industry," *Symposium on Premenstrual Tension, International Record of Medicine,* November 1953.

S. Charles Freed. "History and Causation of Premenstrual Tension," in *Symposium on Premenstrual Tension, International Record of Medicine,* November 1953.

J.P. Greenhill. "Treatment of Premenstrual Tension by Electrolytes," *Symposium on Premenstrual Tension, International Record of Medicine,* November 1953.

Leon Israel. "The Clinical Pattern and Etiology of Premenstrual Tension," in *Symposium on Premenstrual Tension, International Record of Medicine,* November 1953.

Lamb et al. "Premenstrual Tension: E.E.G., Hormonal, and Psychiatric Evaluation." *American Journal of Psychiatry,* 109: 840-848, May 1953.

Joseph H. Morton, ed. *Symposium on Premenstrual Tension, International Record of Medicine,* November 1953.

Joseph H. Morton. "Treatment of Premenstrual Tension," *Symposium on Premenstrual Tension, International Record of Medicine,* November 1953.

Edward L. Suarez-Murais. "The Psychophysiologic Syndrome of Premenstrual Tension," *Symposium on Premenstrual Tension, in International Record of Medicine ,* November 1953.

Mukherjee. "Premenstrual Tension: A Critical Study of the Syndrome," *Journal of the Indian Medical Association,* 1954.

Katharina Dalton. "The Similarity of Symptomatology of PMS and Toxaemia," *British Medical Journal,* 1954.

A.B. Hegarty. "Post-Puerperal Recurrent Depression." *British Medical Journal,* 1955.

G.W. Thorne. "Cyclical Edema." *American Journal of Medicine,* 23: 507, 1957.

Erle Henriksen. "The Melancholies of Menstruation or Premenstrual Tension," *Clinical Obstetrics and Gynecology,* 252-259, 1965.

P.W. Adams et al. "Effects of Pyridoxine Hydrochloride (Vitamin B-6) upon Depression Associated with Oral Contraception." *Lancet,* 1: 899-904, April 28, 1973.

International Congress of Psychosomatic Obstetrics and Gynecology, Sixth Annual Session, Berlin, September 1980.

Guy Abraham. "Premenstrual Tension." *Current Problems in Obstetrics and Gynecology.,* III, 12:5-39, April 1981.

Robert Reid and S.S.C. Yen. "Premenstrual Syndrome." *American Journal of Obstetrics and Gynecology*, 139: 85-104, 1981.

Chapter 3 Migraine

Joan Didion. "In Bed" in *The White Album*. New York: Pocket Books, 1978.

Katharina Dalton. "Progesterone Suppositories and Pessaries in the Treatment of Menstrual Migraine." *Headache*, 12,4: 151-159, January 1973.

Katharina Dalton. "Do It Yourself." *Migraine News Letter of British Migraine Association*, April 1975.

Katharina Dalton. "Food Intake Prior to a Migraine Attack." *Headache*, 15, 3: 188-193, October 1975.

M.T. Epstein et al. "Migraine and Reproductive Hormones Throughout the Menstrual Cycle." *The Lancet*, 543-549, March 8, 1975.

Chapter 4 Epilepsy

Fyodor Dostoevsky. *The Idiot*. New York: Signet Classics, 1969.

Alfred Gordon. "Epilepsy in its Relation to Menstrual Periods." *New York Medical Journal*, XC, 16: 733-736, October 16, 1909.

John Logothetis et al. "The Role of Estrogens in Catmenial Exacerbation of Epilepsy." *Neurology*, 352-360, date TK.

R.H. Mattson et al. "Psychophysiological Precipitants of Seizures in Epileptics." *Neurology*, 20: 407, 1970.

R.H. Mattson et al. "Precipitating and Inhibiting Factors in Epilepsy: A Statistical Study." *Epilepsia*, 15: 271-272, 1974.

Susan Hall. "Treatment of Menstrual Epilepsy with Progesterone Only Contraceptives." *Epilepsia*, 18,2: 235-236, 1977.

Trevor R.P. Price. "Temporal Lobe Epilepsy as a Premenstrual Behavioral Syndrome." *Biological Psychiatry*, 15,6: 957-963, 1980.

Interview with Dr. Allen Hauser, assistant professor of neurology and public health, Columbia University and assistant director of Columbia's Sergievsky Center for the study of epilepsy and cerebral palsy.

Chapter 5 Mood Swings and Depression

Hans Christian Andersen. "The Snow Queen," in *Fairy Tales*. New York: Grosset and Dunlap, 1981.

Dr. Myrna Weissman, quoted in Maggie Scarf's *Unfinished Business*, New York: Ballantine Books, 1981, pp. 594-601.

Constance Berry and Frederick L. McGuire. "Menstrual Distress and Acceptance of Sexual Role," *American Journal of Obstetrics and Gynecology,* 114:1, September 1, 1972, p. 84.

Paula Weideger. *Menstruation and Menopause,* op.cit.

Karl Menninger, quoted in Weideger.

George S. Glass et al. "Psychiatric Emergency Related to the Menstrual Cycle." *American Journal of Psychiatry,* 128,6: 61, December 1971.

Natalie Shainess. "Psychiatric Evaluation of Premenstrual Tension." *New York State Journal of Medicine,* 3573-3579, November 15, 1962.

Katharina Dalton. "Menstruation and Accidents." *British Medical Journal,* 1425-1426, November 12, 1960.

Walter R. Gove. "Sex Differences in Mental Illness Among Adult Men and Women." *Social Science and Medicine,* 12B: 187-198, 1978.

Meir Steiner and Bernard J. Carroll. "The Psychobiology of Premenstrual Dysphoria: Review of Theories and Treatments." *Psychoneuroendocrinology,* 2: 321-335, 1977.

Phyllis Chesler. *Women and Madness*. New York: Avon Books, 1975.

Brian Moore. *I Am Mary Dunne,* op.cit. pp. 211, 215 and 217.

Chapter 6 Eating Disorders

Mary Gordon. *Final Payments*. New York: Ballantine Books, 1979.

Hilde Bruch. *Eating Disorders*. New York: Basic Books Inc., 1973.

Stuart Smith and Cynthia Sauder. "Food Cravings, Depression, and Premenstrual Problems." *Psychosomatic Medicine,* XXXI, 4: 281-286, 1969.

H. Sutherland and I. Stewart. "A Critical Analysis of the Premenstrual Syndrome." *The Lancet.*

J.N. Fortin et al. "Psychosomatic Approach to Premenstrual Tension Syndrome." *CMAJ,* 79: 978, 1958.

J.H. Morton et al. "A Clinical Study of Premenstrual Tension." *American Journal of Obstetrics and Gynecology,* 65: 1182, 1953.

Mara Selvini Palazzoli. *Self-Starvation.* New York: Aronson, 1978.

Sheila MacLeod. op. cit., pp.56-57.

Chapter 7 Problems with Alcohol and Drugs

Joyce Rebeta-Burditt. *The Cracker Factory.* New York: Bantam Books, 1978.

Marian Sandmaier. *The Invisible Alcoholics.* New York: McGraw-Hill Inc., 1981.

Edith S. Gomberg. "Problems with Alcohol and Other Drugs." *Gender and Disordered Behavior.* New York: Brunner/Mazel, 1979.

Myron L. Belfer et al. "Alcoholism in Women." *Archives of General Psychiatry,* 25: 540-544, December 1971.

Jean Kinney and Gwen Leaton. *Understanding Alcohol.* St. Louis: The Mosely Press, 1982.

Interview with Dr. Michael Murphy, president of the Bay Area Comprehensive Alcoholic Program, Boston, Mass.

Chapter 8 It Runs in Families

References drawn from our practice and interviews with patients.

Martha K. McClintock. "Menstrual Synchrony and Suppression." *Nature,* 229,244: 5282, 1971.

Section III Living With PMS

Chapter 9 Strains on Relationships

References drawn from our practice and interviews with patients.

Chapter 10 On the Job

Studs Terkel. *Working*. New York: Avon Books, 1975.

References from our practice and interviews with patients.

Chapter 11 Striking Out

Victoria Lincoln. A Private Disgrace, Lizzie Borden by *Daylight*. New York: G.P. Putnam's Sons, 1967.

Ann Jones. *Women Who Kill*. New York: Fawcett Columbine, 1981.

Katharina Dalton. "Cyclical Criminal Acts in Premenstrual Syndrome." *The Lancet*, 1070-1071, November 15, 1980.

D.P. Ellis and P. Austin. "Menstruation and Aggressive Behavior in a Correctional Center for Women." *Journal of Criminal Law, Criminology and Police Science*, 62: 388-395, 1971.

P. Epps. "Women Shoplifters in Holloway Prison," in *Shoplifting*, ed. by T.C.N. Gibbens and J. Prince. London: Institute for the Study and Treatment of Delinquency, 1962, pp. 132-145.

Katharina Dalton. "Children's Hospital Admissions and Mother's Menstruation." *British Medical Journal*, 27-28, April 4, 1970.

P.T. d'Orban and J. Dalton. "Violent Crime and the Menstrual Cycle." *Psychological Medicine*, 10: 353-359, 1980.

Christine Crawford. *Mommie Dearest*. New York: Berkley Books, 1981.

C. Henry Kempre and Ray E. Helfer. *Helping the Battered Child and His Family*. Philadelphia and Toronto: J.B. Lippincott Company, 1982.

Chapter 12 Suicide Attempts

Leslie Farber. *The Ways of the Will*. New York: Basic Books, 1966.

Boris Pasternak. *An Essay in Autobiography*. TKTK.

Cesare Pavese. *This Business of Living*, translated by A. E. Murch. London and Toronto: 1961.

Rollo May. *Power and Innocence*. New York: Delta Books, 1981.

Sylvia Plath. *The Collected Poems*. New York: Harper and Row, 1982.

Sylvia Plath. *The Bell Jar*. New York: Bantam Books, 1972.

Sylvia Plath. *The Journals of Sylvia Plath*. New York: Dial Press, 1982.

A. Alvarez. *The Savage God — A Study of Suicide*. New York: Random House, 1970.

Richard D. Wetzel et al. "Premenstrual Symptoms in Self-Referrals to a Suicide Prevention Service." *British Journal of Psychiatry*, 119: 525-526, 1971.

Richard D. Wetzel and J.N. McClure Jr. "Suicide and the Menstrual Cycle." *Comprehensive Psychiatry*, 13,4: 369, 1972.

Dorothy Parker. "You Might As Well Live" in *The Portable Dorothy Parker*. New York: The Viking Press, 1973.

Walter R. Gove. "Sex, Marital Status and Suicide." *Journal of Health and Social Behavior*, 13: 204-213, June 1972.

Section IV Female Complaints

Chapter 13 The Pill

Richard I. Shader and Jane I. Ohly. "Premenstrual Tension, Femininity and Sexual Drive." *Medical Aspects of Human Sexuality*, April 1970.

J.R. Udry and N. Morris. "Distribution of Coitus in the Menstrual Cycle." *Nature*, 220:593, November 1968.

Chapter 14 Pregnancy

Sandra McPherson. "Pregnancy," in *A Book of Women Poets*, edited by Aliki Barnstone and Willis Barnstone. New York: Schocken Books, 1980, p. 556.

Katharina Dalton. "Progesterone in Toxaemia of Pregnancy." *Medical World*, December 1955.

Katharina Dalton. "Ante-natal Progesterone and Intelligence." *British Journal of Psychiatry*, 144: 1377-1382, 1968.

Katharina Dalton. "Controlled Trials in the Prophylactic Value of Progesterone in the Treatment of Pre-Eclamptic Toxaemia." *Journal of Obstetrics and Gynaecology* (U.K.), 69: 463-468, June 1962.

Mohamed B. Sammour et al. "Progesterone Therapy in Pre-Eclamptic Toxaemia." *Acta Obstetrica Gynecologica Scandinavica*, 54: 195-202, 1975.

Pentti K. Siiteri. "Progesterone and Maintenance of Pregnancy: Is Progesterone Nature's Immunosuppressant?" *Annals of the New York Academy of Science*, 286:434-445, March 1979.

Chapter 15 Post-Partum Depression

Doris Lessing. *A Proper Marriage*. New York: Plume Books, 1970.

Katharina Dalton. "Prospective Study into Puerperal Depression." *British Journal of Psychiatry*, 118: 689-692, 1971.

A.B. Hegarty. "Post-Puerperal Recurrent Depression." *British Medical Journal*, 637-640, March 12, 1955.

Brice Pitt. "Maternity Blues." *British Journal of Psychiatry*, 122: 431-433, 1973.

C. Dean and R.E. Kendell. "The Symptomatology of Puerperal Illnesses." *British Journal of Psychiatry*, 139: 128, 1981.

Brice Pitt. "Psychiatric Illness Following Childbirth." 409-415.

Amos Weiner. "Childbirth-Related Psychiatric Illness." *Comprehensive Psychiatry*, 23,2: 143-154, March/April 1982.

Willis H. Bower and Mark D. Altschule. "Use of Progesterone in the Treatment of Post-Partum Psychosis." *The New England Journal of Medicine*, 254,4: 157-160, January 26, 1956.

Chapter 16 Sterilization

Montagu G. Barker. "Psychiatric Illness After Hysterectomy." *British Medical Journal*, 91-95, April 13, 1968.

C.T. Backstrom et al. "Persistence of Symptoms of Premenstrual Tension in Hysterectomized Women." *British Journal of Obstetrics and Gynaecology,* 88: 530-536, 1981.

Section V Life Phases

Chapter 17 Adolescence

Carson McCullers. *The Member of the Wedding.* New York: Bantam Books, 1950.

Erik Erikson. *Identity Youth and Crisis.* New York and London: W.W. Norton and Company, 1968.

Janet W. McArthur. "Common Menstrual Disorders in the Adolescent Girl." *Clinical Pediatrics,* 3,11: 663, 1964.

Mark D. Altschule and Jacob Brem. "Periodic Psychosis of Puberty." *American Journal of Psychiatry,* 119: 1176-1177, 1963.

Fred S. Berlin et al. "Periodic Psychosis of Puberty: A Case Report." *American Journal of Psychiatry,* 139,1: 119-120, January 1982.

Jagdish S. Teja. "Periodic Psychosis of Puberty: A Longitudinal Case Study." *The Journal of Nervous and Mental Disease,* 162,1: 52-57, 1976.

Rose E. Frisch. "Critical Weights, a Critical Body Composition, Menarche and the Maintenance of the Menstrual Cycle," in *Biosocial Interrelation in Population Adaptation.* The Hague: Mouton & Company.

Rose E. Frisch and Roger Revell. "Height and Weight at Menarche and a Hypothesis of Menarche." *Archives of Diseases in Childhood,* 46, 249: 695, 1971.

Rose E. Frisch, Roger Revell and Sole Cook. "Components of Weight at Menarche and the Initiation of the Adolescent Growth Spurt in Girls." *Human Biology,* 45,3: 469, 1973.

Chapter 18 The Twenties and Thirties

Gail Sheehy. *Passages.* New York: E.P. Dutton Inc., 1974.

Chapter 19 The Forties

Carl Jung. *Modern Man in Search of a Soul*. New York and London: Harvest Books, 1933.

Chapter 20 Menopause and Post-Menopause

Doris Lessing. *The Summer Before the Dark*. New York: Bantam Books. 1974.

Elizabeth Barrett Browning. *Sonnets from the Portuguese*.

William Faulkner. A Light in August. New York: Random House, 1967.

William Shakespeare. *The Tragedy of Hamlet, Prince of Denmark*. New York: Washington Square Press, 1958.

Sonja M. McKinlay and Margot Jefferys. "The Menopausal Syndrome." *British Journal of Preventive and Social Medicine*, 28, 2: 108, 1974.

Section VI The PMS Prescription

Chapter 21 Do You Have PMS?

Material developed for our centers.

Chapter 22 The PMS Diet

Guy Abraham. "Nutritional Factors in the Etiology of the Premenstrual Tension Syndrome." *Journal of Reproductive Medicine*. 28: 446, 1983.

Jane Brody. Jane Brody's *Nutrition Book*. New York and London: W.W. Norton and Company, 1981.

Adele Davis. *Let's Get Well*. New York: Harcourt Brace and World Inc., 1965.

Mildred S. Seelig. "The Requirement of Magnesium by the Normal Adult." *American Journal of Clinical Nutrition*, 14: 342-390, June 1964.

Chapter 23 Vitamin Therapy

Guy Abraham. "Nutritional Factors in the Etiology of the Premenstrual Tension Syndrome." *Journal of Reproductive Medicine*. 28: 446, 1983.

Guy Abraham. "Premenstrual Tension." *Current Problems in Obstetrics and Gynecology*, III, 12: 5-39, April 1981.

Morton S. Biskind. "Nutritional Deficiency in the Etiology of Menorrhagia, Metrohagia, Cystic Mastitis and Premenstrual Tension, Treatment with Vitamin B Complex." *Journal of Clinical Endocrinology and Metabolism*, 3: 227-234, 1943.

Clement G. Martin. *Low Blood Sugar: The Hidden Menace of Hypoglycemia*. New York: Arco Publishing Inc., 1969.

Chapter 24 Getting Physical

Kenneth H. Cooper. *Aerobics*. New York: Bantam Books, 1980.

Chapter 25 Managing Stress

Hans Selye. *The Physiology and Pathology of Exposure to Stress*. Montreal, Canada: Acta Inc., 1950.

Hans Selye. *The Stress of Life*. New York: McGraw-Hill Inc., 1956.

Herbert Benson. *The Relaxation Response*. New York: Avon Books, 1975.

Thomas Holmes and Richard Rahe. "The Social Readjustment Rating Scale." *Journal of Psychosomatic Research*, 11: 213, 1967.

Chapter 26 The Progesterone Story

See bibliography for extensive listing of all related articles. Following are cited in order they appear in text.

S.S.C. Yen et al. "Hormonal Relationships During the Menstrual Cycle." *Journal of the American Medical Association*, 211, 9: 1513-1517, March 2, 1970.

Robert L. Reid and S.S.C. Yen. "Premenstrual Syndrome." *American Journal of Obstetrics and Gynecology*, 139: 85-104, 1981.

Willard M. Allen. "Progesterone: How Did the Name Originate?" *Southern Medical Journal*, 63, 10: 1151-1155, October 1970.

Willard M. Allen. "Recollections of My Life With Progesterone." *Gynecological Investigations*, 5: 142-182, 1974.

Katharina Dalton. "A Guide to Premenstrual Syndrome and Its Treatment." K. Dalton, London, 1981.

Katharina Dalton. "Comparative Trials of New Oral Progestogenic Compounds in Treatment of Premenstrual Syndrome." *British Medical Journal*, 1307-1309, December 12, 1959.

Doyle W. Frank. "Mammary Tumors and Serum Hormones in the Bitch Treated with Medroxyprogesterone Acetate or Progesterone for Four Years." *Fertility and Sterility*, 31,3: 340-346, March 1979.

Linda Cowan et al. "Breast Cancer Incidence in Women With a History of Progesterone Deficiency." *American Journal of Epidemiology*, 114,2: 209-217, 1981.

Joseph Gilman. "Nature of Subjective Reaction Evoked in Women by Progesterone with Special Reference to the Problem of Premenstrual Tension." *Journal of Clinical Endocrinology and Metabolism*, 2: 156, 1942.

L.A. Gray. "The Use of Progesterone in Nervous Tension States." *Southern Medical Journal*, 1004-1010, September 1941.

David A. Hamburg. "Effects of Progesterone on Behavior," in *Endocrines and the Central Nervous System*, Levine and Rachkiel eds. Baltimore: Williams & Wilkins Company, 1966.

David A. Hamburg and Donald T. Lunde. "Sex Hormones in the Development of Sex Differences in Human Behavior," in *The Development of Sex Differences*, Eleanor E. Maccoby ed. Stanford, Calif.: Stanford University Press, 1966.

Arthur Herbst et al. "The Effects of Local Progesterone on Stilbestrol-Associated Vaginal Adenosis." *American Journal of Obstetrics and Gynecology*, 607-615, March 1, 1974.

IARC Monograph. "Evaluation of the Carcinogenic Risk of Chemicals to Man: Sex Hormones." Lyon, February 4-11, 1974, vol. 6.

Mary-Claire King. "Risk Factors in Breast Cancer," a review of *Hormones and Breast Cancer, in Science*, 214: 1122-1123, December 9, 1981.

Sophia J. Kleegman and Sherwin A. Kaufman. "The Endocrines Concerned with Menstruation and Infertility," in *Infertility in Women*. Philadelphia: F.A. Davis, 1966.

Frederick Naftolin and George Tolis. "Neuroendocrine Regulation of the Menstrual Cycle." *Clinical Obstetrics and Gynecology*, 21,1: 17-29, March 1978.

Gwyneth A. Sampson. "Premenstrual Syndrome: A Double-Blind Controlled Trial of Progesterone and Placebo." *British Journal of Psychiatry*, 135:209-215, 1979.

Gwyneth A. Sampson. "An Appraisal of the Role of Progesterone in the Therapy of Premenstrual Syndrome" in *The Premenstrual Syndrome*, ed. by P.A. van Keep. Lancaster, England: MTP Press Ltd., Falcon House International Medical Publishers, 1981, pp.51-69.

Mona Shangold. "The Relationship Between Long-Distance Running, Plasma Progesterone, and Luteal Phase Length." *Fertility and Sterility*, 31,130: 607-608, 1979.

Pentti K. Siiteri. "Progesterone and Maintenance of Pregnancy: Is Progesterone Nature's Immunosuppressant?" *Annals of the New York Academy of Science*, 286: 434-445, March 1979.

Leon Speroff and Raymond Vande Wiele. "Regulation of the Human Menstrual Cycle." *American Journal of Obstetrics and Gynecology*, 109,2: 232-247, January 15, 1971.

Bruce V. Stadel. "Oral Contraceptives and Cardiovascular Disease." *New England Journal of Medicine*, 612-677, September 10, 1981.

Paul Beck. "Effects of Progestins on Glucose and Lipid Metabolism." *Annals of the New York Academy of Science*, 286: 343-355, March 1979.

Allan C. Barnes and Irving Rothchild. "Experimental Use of Intravenously Administered Progesterone in Advanced Cases of Cervical Carcinoma." *Obstetrics and Gynecology*, 1,2: 147-155, February 1953.

Anne Colston Wentz. "Assessment of Estrogen and Progestin Therapy in Gynecology and Obstetrics." *Clinical Obstetrics and Gynecology*, 20,2:461-480, June 1977.

M.I. Whitehead et al. "Absorption and Metabolism of Oral Progesterone." *Gynecology*, 36,1: 32-33, 1981.

Section VII The Broader View

Chapter 27 Fame Is No Protection

Carolly Erikson. *Bloody Mary*. New York: Doubleday and Company Inc., 1978.

Louis Auchincloss. *Persons of Consequence, Queen Victoria and Her Circle*. New York: Random House, 1979.

Alison Plowden. *Marriage With My Kingdom*. New York: Stein and Day, 1977.

Herbert Tingsten. *Victoria and the Victorians*. New York: Delacorte Press, 1972.

Len Ortzen. *Imperial Venus*. New York: Stein and Day, 1974.

Ruth Painter Randall. *Mary Lincoln — Biography of a Marriage*. Boston: Little Brown and Company, 1953.

W.A. Evans. *Mrs. Abraham Lincoln — A Study of Her Personality and Her Influence on Lincoln*. New York: Alfred A. Knopf Inc., 1932.

Jean Strouse. *Alice James*. New York: Bantam Books, 1982.

Arianna Stassinopoulos. *Maria Callas*. New York: Ballantine Books, 1982.

Christopher Finch. *Rainbow*. New York: Grosset & Dunlap, 1975.

Edward Butscher. *Sylvia Plath: Method and Madness*. New York: Washington Square Press, 1976.

Sylvia Plath. *The Bell Jar*. op. cit.

Sylvia Plath. *The Collected Poems*. op. cit.

Sylvia Plath. *The Journals*. op. cit.

A. Alvarez. *The Savage God*. op. cit.

Chapter 28 The Defense Pleads PMS

Aleta Wallach and Larry Rubin. "The Premenstrual Syndrome and Criminal Responsibility." *UCLA Law Review*, 19: 209-312, 1971.

Katharina Dalton. "Cyclical Criminal Acts in Premenstrual Syndrome." op.cit.

Katharina Dalton. "Legal Implications of PMS." *World Medicine*, 93-94, April 17, 1982.

Diana Brahams. "Premenstrual Syndrome: A Disease of the Mind?" *The Lancet*, 1238-1240, November 28, 1981.

Diana Brahams. "Rejection of Premenstrual Syndrome as a Defence in English Law." *The Lancet*, 1134-1135, May 15, 1982.

P.T. d'Orban. "Premenstrual Syndrome." *The Lancet*, ii, 1413.

Julie Horney. "Menstrual Cycles and Criminal Responsibility." *Law and Human Behavior*, 2,1: 25-36, 1978.

Kenneth K. Fukunaga et al. "Insanity Plea." *Law and Human Behavior*, 5,4: 325-328, 1981.

Peter Arenella. "The Diminished Capacity and Diminished Responsibility Defenses: Two Children of a Doomed Marriage." *Columbia Law Review*, 77, 6: 827-863, October 1977.

R.D. Mackay. "Non-Organic Automatism — Some Recent Developments." *The Criminal Law Review*, 350-361, 1978.

Geraldine Brotherton. "Post-Traumatic Stress Disorder — Opening Pandora's Box?" *New England Law Review*, 17,1: 91-117, 1981.

Chapter 29 *Making Progress*

References to materials from our center.

Telephone interview with Susan Brownmiller.

Selected Bibliography

Abraham, Guy, E. et al. "Evaluation of Ovulation and Corpus Luteum Function in Using Measurements of Plasma Progesterone." *Obstetrics and Gynecology*, 44: 522, 1974.

Abraham, G.E., and Hargrove, J.T. "Effect of Vitamin B-6 on Premenstrual Symptomatology in Women with Premenstrual Tension Syndrome: A Double Crossover Study." *Infertility*, 3: 155-165, 1980.

Abraham, G.E. "Nutritional Factors in the Etiology of the Premenstrual Tension Syndrome." *Journal of Reproductive Medicine*, 28: 446, 1983.

Abraham, G.E. "Premenstrual Tension." *Current Problems in Obstetrics and Gynecology*, III, 12: 5-39, April 1981.

Abraham, G.E., and Lubran, M.M. "Serum and Red Cell Magnesium Levels in Patients with Premenstrual Tensions." *American Journal of Applied Nutrition*, 34: 4, 1982.

Ackerknecht, Erwin, H. "The History of Psychosomatic Medicine." *Psychological Medicine*, 12: 17-24, 1982.

Allen, Willard M. "Progesterone: How Did the Name Originate?" *Southern Medical Journal*, 63, 10: 1151-1155, October 1970.

Allen, Willard M. "Recollections of My Life With Progesterone." *Gynecological Investigations*, 5: 142-182, 1974.

Altschule, Mark D., and Brem, Jacob. "Periodic Psychosis of Puberty." *American Journal of Psychiatry*, 119: 1176-1178, 1963.

Alvarez, A. *The Savage God—A Study of Suicide*. New York: Random House, 1970.

American Psychiatric Association. *Diagnostic and Statistical Manual of Mental Disorders*, third edition. Washington, D.C., APA, 1980.

Andersen, Hans Christian. "The Snow Queen," in *Fairy Tales*. New York: Grosset and Dunlap, 1981.

Appleby, B.P. "A Study of Premenstrual Tension in General Practice." *British Medical Journal*, 1: 391, February 1960.

Arenella, Peter. "The Diminished Capacity and Diminished Responsibility Defenses: Two Children of a Doomed Marriage." *Columbia University Law Review,* 77, 6: 827-863, October 1977.

Auchincloss, Louis. *Persons of Consequence, Queen Victoria and Her Circle.* New York: Random House, 1979.

Backstrom, C.T. et al. "Persistence of Symptoms of Premenstrual Tension in Hysterectomized Women." *British Journal of Obstetrics and Gynaecology,* 88:530-536, 1981.

Baker, H.W.G. et al. "Rhythms in the Secretion of Gonadotropins and Gonadal Steroids." *Journal of Steroidal Biochemistry,* 6: 793, 1975.

Ballantine, R. *Diet and Nutrition: A Holistic Approach.* Honesdale, Pennsylvania: Himalayan International Institute, 1978.

Barker, Montagu G. "Psychiatric Illness after Hysterectomy." *British Medical Journal,* April 13, 1968, 91-95.

Barnes, Allan C. and Rothchild, Irving. "Experimental Use of Intravenously Administered Progesterone in Advanced Cases of Cervical Carcinoma." *Obstetrics and Gynecology.* 1, 2: 147-155, February 1953.

Barnes, A.C., ed. *Progesterone.* Augusta, Michigan: Brook Lodge Press, 1961.

Barton, D.H. "The Conformation of the Steroid Nucleus." *Experientia,* VI (8): 316-320, 1950.

Beck, Paul. "Effects of Progestins on Glucose and Lipid Metabolism." *Annals of the New York Academy of Science,* 286: 434-455, March 1979.

Beecher, Henry K. "Relationship of Significance of Wound to Pain Experienced." *Journal of the American Medical Association,* 161,7: 1609-1613, August 25, 1956.

Belfer, Myron L. et al. "Alcoholism in Women." *Archives of General Psychiatry,* 25: 540-544, December 1971.

Bell, Donald H. *Being a Man — The Paradox of Masculinity.* Brattleboro, Vt.: The Lewis Publishing Company, 1982.

Benedict, Ruth. *Patterns of Culture*. Boston: Houghton Mifflin, 1934.

Benson, Ralph C., ed. *Current Obstetric and Gynecologic Diagnosis and Treatment*. Los Altos, Calif.: Lange Medical Publications, fourth edition, 1976.

Berlin, Fred S. et al. "Periodic Psychosis of Puberty. A Case Report." *American Journal of Psychiatry,* 139, 1: 119-120. January 1982.

Berry, Constance and McGuire, Frederick L. "Menstrual Distress and Acceptance of Sexual Role." *American Journal of Obstetrics and Gynecology,* 114: 84, September 1972.

Bertioli, A. et al. "Differences in Insulin Receptors Between Men and Menstruating Women and Influence of Sex Hormones on Insulin Binding During the Menstrual Cycle." *Journal of Clinical Endocrinology and Metabolics,* 50:246-250, 1980.

Bettelheim, Bruno. *Symbolic Wounds*. New York: Collier Books, 1962.

Billig, Harvey E. Jr. and Spaulding, C. Arthur Jr. "Hyperinsulinism of Menses." *Industrial Medicine,* July 1947, 336-339.

Billig, Harvey E. Jr. "The Role of Premenstrual Tension in Industry." *International Record of Medicine,* 166, 11: 487-491, November 1953.

Biskind, Morton S. "Nutritional Deficiency in the Etiology of Menorrhagia, Metrohagia, Cystic Mastilis and Premenstrual Tension, Treatment with Vitamin B Complex." *Journal of Clinical Endocrinology and Metabolism,* 3: 227-234, 1943.

Boyd, A.E., Reichlin, S. et al. "Galactorrhea-Amenorrhea Syndrome: Diagnosis and Therapy." *Annals of Internal Medicine,* 87: 165, 1977.

Brahams, Diana. "Medicine and the Law: Premenstrual Syndrome — a Disease of the Mind?" *The Lancet,* November 28, 1981, 1238-1240.

Brahams, Diana. "Rejection of Premenstrual Syndrome as a Defence in English Law." *The Lancet,* 1134-1135, May 15, 1982.

Breuer, Josef and Sigmund Freud, *Studies on Hysteria, translated by James Strachey*. New York: Basic Books Inc., 1982.

Briscoe, Monica. "Sex Differences in Psychological Well-Being," monograph supplement in *Psychological Medicine*. Cambridge, London and New York: Cambridge University Press, 1982.

Brotherton, Geraldine L. "Post-Traumatic Stress Disorder — Opening Pandora's Box?" *New England Law Review*, 17, 1: 91-117, 1981.

Bruch, Hilde. *Eating Disorders*. New York: Basic Books Inc., 1973.

Brush, M. "Therapy for the Woman with Premenstrual Syndrome." *Mims*, April 1, 1982, 7-31.

Bullough, Vern and Voght, Martha. "Women, Menstruation, and Nineteenth-Century Medicine." *Bulletin of Historical Medicine*, 47: 66-82, 1973.

Burkhart, Kathryn. *Women in Prison*. New York: Doubleday and Company, 1973.

Butscher, Edward. *Sylvia Plath: Method and Madness*. New York: Washington Square Press, 1977.

Campbell, Joseph, ed. *The Portable Jung*. New York: Penguin Books, 1976.

Carsten, Mary E. "Hormonal Regulation of Myometrial Calcium Transport." *Gynecological Investigations*, 5:269-275, 1974.

Chadwick, Mary. *The Psychology of Menstruation* (Monograph 56). Washington, D.C.: Nervous and Mental Diseases Publishing Company, 1932.

Chesler, Phyllis. *Women and Madness*. New York: Avon Books, 1972.

Chez, R.A. "Proceedings of the Symposium: Progesterone, Progestins, and Fetal Development." *Fertility and Sterility*, 30: 16, 1978.

Clarke, Edward H. *Sex in Education*, 1873.

Colquhoun, W.P. ed. *Biological Rhythms and Human Performance*. London and New York: Academic Press, 1971.

Colt, Edward W.D. et al. "The Effect of Running on Plasma B-Endorphin." *Life Science*, 28, 1637, 1982.

Cooper, Kenneth H. *Aerobics*. New York: Bantam Books, 1980.

Cowan, Linda et al. "Breast Cancer Incidence in Women With a History of Progesterone Deficiency." *American Journal of Epidemiology*, 114, 2: 209-217, 1981.

Crawford, Christine. *Mommie Dearest*. New York: Berkley Books, 1981.

Crawfurd, Raymond. "Superstitions of Menstruation." *The Lancet*, December 18, 1915.

Croucher, M.J. et al. "Anticonvulsant Action of Excitatory Amino Acid Antagonists." *Science*, 216: 899-901, May 21, 1982.

Dalton, Katharina and Greene, Raymond. "The Premenstrual Syndrome." *British Medical Journal*, 1071-1016, May 9, 1953.

Dalton, Katharina. "Similarity of Symptomatology of Premenstrual Syndrome and Toxaemia of Pregnancy and Their Response to Progesterone." *British Medical Journal*, 1071-1076, November 6, 1954.

Dalton, Katharina. "Progesterone in Toxaemia of Pregnancy." *Medical World*, 1-3, December 1955.

Dalton, Katharina. "Comparative Trials of New Oral Progestogenic Compounds in Treatment of Premenstrual Syndrome." *British Medical Journal*, 1307-1309, December 12, 1959.

Dalton, Katharina. "Effects of Menstruation on Schoolgirls' Weekly Work." *British Medical Journal*, 326-328, January 30, 1960.

Dalton, Katharina. "Menstruation and Accidents." *British Medical Journal*, 1425-1426, November 12, 1960.

Dalton, Katharina. "Controlled Trials in the Prophylactic Value of Progesterone in the Treatment of Pre-Eclamptic Toxaemia." *Journal of Obstetrics and Gynaecology*, 69: 463-468, June 1962.

Dalton, Katharina. "A Guide to Premenstrual Syndrome and Its Treatment." K. Dalton, London, 1981.

Dalton, Katharina. "Menstruation and Examinations." *The Lancet*, 1386-1388, December 28, 1968.

Dalton, Katharina. "Ante-Natal Progesterone and Intelligence." *British Journal of Psychiatry*, 114: 1377-1382, 1968.

Dalton, Katharina. "Children's Hospital Admissions and Mother's Menstruation." *British Medical Journal*, 27-28, April 4, 1970.

Dalton, Katharina. "Prospective Study into Puerperal Depression." *British Journal of Psychiatry,* 113: 689-692, 1971.

Dalton, Katharina. "Progesterone Suppositories and Pessaries in the Treatment of Menstrual Migraine." *Headache,* 12, 4: 151-159, January 1973.

Dalton, Katharina. "Food Intake Prior to a Migraine Attack — Study of 2,313 Spontaneous Attacks." *Headache,* 15, 3: 188-193, October 1975.

Dalton, Katharina. "Cyclical Criminal Acts in Premenstrual Syndrome." *The Lancet,* 1070-1071, November 15, 1980.

Davis, Adele. *Let's Get Well.* New York: Harcourt Brace and World Inc., 1965.

deBeauvoir, Simone. *The Second Sex.* New York: Alfred A. Knopf, 1952.

Debrovner, C., ed. *Premenstrual Tension.* New York: Human Sciences Press, 1982.

Delaney, Janice, et al. *The Curse, A Cultural History of Menstruation.* New York: E.P. Dutton and Company Inc., 1976.

Dempsey, M.E. "Regulation of Steroid Biosynthesis." *Annual Review of Biochemistry,* 44: 967, 1975.

Deutsch, Helene. *The Psychology of Women, volumes I and II.* New York: Grune and Stratton, 1944.

Diabetes, "ADA Statement on Hypoglycemia." *Diabetes,* 22: 137, 1973.

Didion, Joan. *The White Album.* New York: Pocket Books, 1978.

Doering, C.H. et al. "A Cycle of Plasma Testosterone in the Human Male." *Journal of Clinical Endocrinology and Metabolism,* 40: 492, 1975.

d'Orban, P.T. and Dalton, J. "Violent Crime and the Menstrual Cycle." *Psychological Medicine,* 10: 353-359, 1980.

Dostoevsky, Fyodor. *The Idiot.* New York: Signet Classics, 1969.

Douglas, Mary. *Purity and Danger: An Analysis of Concepts of Pollution and Taboo*. Baltimore, Md.: Penguin Books, 1970.

Duff, David. *Albert and Victoria*. London: Ludgate House, 1972.

Ehrenreich, Barbara and English, Deirdre. *Complaints and Disorders, The Sexual Politics of Sickness*. Old Westbury, New York: The Feminist Press, 1973.

Eichner, E. and Waltner, C. "Premenstrual Tension." *Medical Times*, 83: 771, 1955.

Eisenberg, L. "The Search for Care." *Daedalus*, 106: 235-246, 1977.

Ellis, D.P. and Austin, P. "Menstruation and Aggressive Behavior in a Correctional Center for Women." *Journal of Criminal Law, Criminology and Police Science*, 62: 388-395, 1971.

Endo, M. et al. "Periodic Psychosis Recurring in Association With the Menstrual Cycle." *Journal of Clinical Psychiatry*, 39: 456-466, 1978.

Engel, G.W. "The Need For a New Medical Model: A Challenge for Biomedicine." *Science*, 196: 129-136, 1977.

Epps, P. "Women Shoplifters in Holloway Prison," in *Shoplifting*, ed. by T.C.N. Gibbens and J. Prince. London: Institute for the Study and Treatment of Delinquency, 1962.

Epstein, M.T. et al. "Migraine and Reproductive Hormones Through the Menstrual Cycle." *The Lancet*, March 8, 1975, 543-547.

Erikson, Carolly. *Bloody Mary*. New York: Doubleday and Company Inc., 1978.

Erikson, Erik H. *Identity Youth and Crisis*. New York and London: W.W. Norton and Company, 1968.

Evans, W.A. *Mrs. Abraham Lincoln — A Study of Her Personality and Her Influence on Lincoln*. New York: Alfred A. Knopf, 1932.

Farber, Leslie. *The Ways of the Will*. New York: Basic Books, 1966.

Ferin, M. et al. eds. *Biorhythms and Human Reproduction*. New York: J. Wiley and Sons, 1974.

Finch, Christopher. *Rainbow*. New York: Grosset & Dunlap, 1975.

Fletcher, Eleanor. *Century of Struggle: The Woman's Rights Movement in the United States.* Cambridge: Harvard University Press, 1959.

Frank, Doyle W. "Mammary Tumors and Serum Hormones in the Bitch Treated With Medroxyprogesterone Acetate or Progesterone for Four Years." *Fertility and Sterility,* 31, 3: 340-346, March 1979.

Frank, Robert T. "Clinical Data Obtained with the Female Sex Hormone Blood Test." *Journal of the American Medical Association,* January 14, 1928.

Frank, Robert T. *The Female Sex Hormone,* New York, 1929.

Frank, Robert T. "Hormonal Causes of Premenstrual Tension." *Archives of Neurology and Psychiatry,* 26: 1053, 1931.

Frantz, A.G. "Prolactin." *New England Journal of Medicine,* 298: 201, 1978.

Frazer, Sir James. *The New Golden Bough.* New York: Mentor Books, 1964.

Freed, S. Charles. "History and Causation of Premenstrual Tension." *International Record of Medicine,* 166: 465-468, November 1953.

Freud, Sigmund. *The Case of Dora and Other Papers.* New York: W.W. Norton & Company, 1952.

Freud, Sigmund. *New Introductory Lectures in Psychoanalysis.* New York: W.W. Norton & Company, 1933.

Freud, Sigmund. *Totem and Taboo.* Harmondsworth, Middlesex: Penguin Books, 1938.

Freud, Sigmund. *Civilization and Its Discontents.* New York: W.W. Norton & Co., 1961.

Friedan, Betty. *The Feminine Mystique.* New York: Dell Publishing Company Inc., 1970.

Frisch, Rose E. "Critical Weights, a Critical Body Composition, Menarche and the Maintenance of the Menstrual Cycle," in *Biosocial Interrelation in Population Adaptation.* The Hague: Mouton & Company. 1974.

Frisch, Rose E. and Roger Revell. "Height and Weight at Menarche and a Hypothesis of Menarche." *Archives of Diseases in Childhood,* 46, 249: 695, 1971.

Frisch, Rose E. et al. "Components of Weight at Menarche and the Initiation of the Adolescent Growth Spurt in Girls." *Human Biology,* 45,3: 469, 1973.

Fukunaga, Kenneth K. "Insanity Plea: Interexaminer Agreement and Concordance of Psychiatric Opinion and Court Verdict." *Law and Human Behavior,* 5: 325-328, November 4, 1981.

Gilman, Joseph. "Nature of Subjective Reaction Evoked in Women by Progesterone with Special Reference to the Problem of Premenstrual Tension." *Journal of Clinical Endocrinology and Metabolism,* 2: 156, 1942.

Glass, George S. et al. "Psychiatric Emergency Related to the Menstrual Cycle." *American Journal of Psychiatry,* 128, 6: 705-711, December 1971.

Gold, J.J. and Josimovich, J.B., eds. *Gynecologic Endocrinology.* New York: Harper & Row, 1980.

Gomberg, Edith S. "Problems with Alcohol and Other Drugs." *Gender and Disordered Behavior.* New York: Brunner/Mazel, 1979.

Gordon, Alfred. "Epilepsy in its Relation to Menstrual Periods." *New York Medical Journal,* XC, 16: 733-736, October 16, 1909.

Gordon, Mary. *Final Payments.* New York: Ballantine Books, 1979.

Gottshalk, Louis A. et al. "Variation in Magnitude of Emotion: A Method Applied to Anxiety and Hostility During Phases of the Menstrual Cycle." *Psychosomatic Medicine,* 24: 300, 1962.

Gove, Walter R. "Sex, Marital Status and Suicide." *Journal of Health and Social Behavior,* June 13, 1972, 204-213.

Gove, Walter R. "Sex Differences in Mental Illness Among Adult Men and Women." *Social Science and Medicine,* 1213: 187-198, 1978.

Gower, D.B. *Steroid Hormones.* Chicago: Year Book Medical Publishers, 1979.

Gray, L. A. "The Use of Progesterone in Nervous Tension States." *Southern Medical Journal,* 1004-1010, September 1941.

Greenblatt, Robert B. "Estrogen Therapy for Postmenopausal Females." *New England Journal of Medicine,* 272: 305, 1963.

Grody, W.W., et al. "Activation, Transformation, and Subunit Structure of Steroid Hormone Receptors." *Endocrine Reviews,* 3: 141-163 1982.

Gump, Frank E. "Common Errors in the Treatment of Benign Breast Lesions." *Drug Therapy,* March, 1982, 67-75.

Hall, Susan M. "Treatment of Menstrual Epilepsy with a Progesterone-Only Oral Contraceptive." *Epilepsia,* 18, 2: 235-236, 1977.

Hamburg, David A. "Effects of Progesterone on Behavior," in *Endocrines and the Central Nervous System,* Levine and Rachkiel eds. Baltimore: Williams & Wilkins Company, 1966.

Hamburg, David A. and Lunde, Donald T. "Sex Hormones in the Development of Sex Differences in Human Behavior," in *The Development of Sex Differences,* Eleanor E. Maccoby ed. Stanford, Calif.: Stanford University Press, 1966.

Hamburg, David A., "Disease Prevention: The Challenge of the Future." *American Journal of Public Health,* 69: 1026-1033, October 1979.

Hamburg, David A. and Trudeau, Michelle B., eds. *Biobehavioral Aspects of Aggression.* New York: Alan R. Liss Inc., 1981.

Hammond, C.B. and Haney, A.F. "Conservative Treatment of Endometriosis." *Fertility and Sterility,* 30: 497, 1978.

Harding, M. Esther. *Woman's Mysteries, Ancient and Modern.* New York: Harper Colophon Books, 1976.

Hart, Ruth Darcy. "Monthly Rhythm of Libido in Married Women." *British Medical Journal,* 1: 1023, 1960.

Haskett, Roger F. et al. "Severe Premenstrual Tension, Delineation of the Syndrome." *Biological Psychiatry,* 15, 1: 121-139, 1980.

Hays, H.R. *The Dangerous Sex.* New York: Putnam, 1965.

Hegarty, A.B. "Post-Puerperal Recurrent Depression." *British Medical Journal,* 637-640, March 12, 1955.

Henriksen, Erle. "The Melancholies of Menstruation, or Premenstrual Tension." *Clinical Obstetrics and Gynecology,* 252-259, 1965.

Herbst, Arthur et al. "The Effects of Local Progesterone on Stilbestrol-Associated Vaginal Adenosis." *American Journal of Obstetrics and Gynecology,* 607-615, March 1, 1974.

Hier, Daniel B. and William F. Crowley. "Spatial Ability in Androgen-Deficient Men." *New England Journal of Medicine,* 1202-1205, May 20, 1982.

Horney, Julie. "Menstrual Cycles and Criminal Responsibility." *Law and Human Behavior,* 2, 1: 25-36, 1978.

Howe, Florence and Ellen Bass, eds. *No More Masks! An Anthology of Poems by Women.* New York: Anchor Press, 1973.

Howe, Julia Ward, ed. *Sex and Education: A Reply to Dr. E.H. Clarke's 'Sex in Education.'* Boston, 1874; New York: Arno Press, 1972.

— IARC Monograph. "Evaluation of the Carcinogenic Risk of Chemicals to Man: Sex Hormones." *Lyon,* vol. 6, February 4-11, 1974.

Icard, S. *La Femme Pendant la Periode Menstruelle.* Paris: Felix Alcan, 1890.

Israel, S. Leon. "Premenstrual Tension." *Journal of the American Medical Association,* 110: 1721-1723, November 21, 1938.

Israel, S. Leon. "The Clinical Pattern and Etiology of Premenstrual Tension." *International Record of Medicine,* 166,11: 469-474, November 1953.

Israel, S. Leon. *Diagnosis and Treatment of Menstrual Disorders and Sterility.* New York: Harper and Row, fifth edition, 1967.

Janiger, Oscar et al. "Cross Cultural Study of Premenstrual Symptoms." *Psychosomatics,* XIII: 226-233, July-August 1972.

Janowsky, David S. et al. "The Curse — Vicissitudes and Variations of the Female Fertility Cycle." *Psychosomatics,* VII: 242, 1966.

Jefferson, J.W. and Marshall, J.R., *Neuropsychiatric Features of Medical Disorders*. New York: Plenum Medical Book Company, 1981.

Johansson, E.D.B. "Depression of the Progesterone Levels in Women Treated with Synthetic Gestagens After Ovulation." *Acta Endocrinologica*, 68: 779, 1971.

Jones, Ann. *Women Who Kill*. New York: Fawcett Columbine, 1981.

Jones, H.W. and Jones, G.S. *Gynecology*. Baltimore: Williams & Wilkins, 1982.

Jordheim, Odd. "The Premenstrual Syndrome." *Acta Obstetrica Gynecologica Scandinavica*, 51: 77, 1972.

Jost, A. "Hormonal Effects on Fetal Development: A Survey." *Clinical Pharmacology and Therapeutics*, 14: 714, 1973.

Jung, Carl C. *Modern Man in Search of a Soul*. New York and London: Harvest Books, 1933.

Jung, Carl C. *Memories, Dreams, Reflections*. New York: Vintage Books, 1965.

Jung, Carl C. *Man and His Symbols*. New York: Dell Publishing Company, 1968.

Jurkowski, J.E. et al. "Ovarian Hormonal Responses to Exercise." *Journal of Applied Physiology*, 44: 109-114, January 1978.

Kane, Alison and Carlson, Eric T. "A Different Drummer: Robert B. Carter and Nineteenth Century Hysteria." *Bulletin of the New York Academy of Medicine*, 58, 6: 519-529, September 1982.

Kapp, M.B. "Prescribing Approved Drugs for Nonapproved Uses: Physicians' Disclosure Obligations to Their Patients." *Law, Medicine and Health Care*, 20-23, October 1981.

Kates, J.E. *Managing Stress*. New York: AMACOM, 1979.

Kempre, C. Henry and Helfer, Ray E. *Helping the Battered Child and His Family*. Philadelphia and Toronto: J.B. Lippincott Company, 1982.

Kerr, G.D. "The Management of the Premenstrual Syndrome." *Current Medical Resident Opinion*, 4 (Supplement 4): 29-34, 1977.

King, Mary-Claire. "Risk Factors in Breast Cancer," a review of *Hormones and Breast Cancer, in Science,* 214: 1122-1123, December 9, 1981.

Kinney, Jean and Leaton, Gwen. *Understanding Alcohol.* St. Louis: The Mosely Press, 1982.

Kleegman, Sophia J. and Kaufman, Sherwin A. "The Endocrines Concerned with Menstruation and Infertility" in *Infertility in Women.* Philadelphia: F.A. Davis, 1966.

Kleinman, A. et al. "Culture, Illness, and Care." *Annals of Internal Medicine,* 88: 251-258, 1978.

Klimt, E.R. et al. "Standardization of the Oral Glucose Tolerance Test." *Diabetes,* 18: 299, 1969.

Kroger, W.S. *Psychosomatic Obstetrics, Gynecology and Endocrinology.* Springfield, Ill.: Charles C Thomas Publisher, 1962.

Lennane, K. Jean and Lennane, R. John. "Alleged Psychogenic Disorders in Women — A Possible Manifestation of Sexual Prejudice." *New England Journal of Medicine,* 288, February 1973.

Lesser, M. *Nutrition and Vitamin Therapy.* New York: Grove Press, 1980.

Lessing, Doris. *A Proper Marriage.* New York: Plume Books, 1970.

Lessing, Doris. *The Summer Before the Dark.* New York: Bantam Books, 1974.

Levi-Strauss, Claude. *Structural Anthropology,* translated by Claire Jacobsen and Brooke Grundfest Schoepf. New York: Basic Books, 1963.

Levine, Lena and Doherty, Beka. *The Menopause.* New York: Random House, 1952.

Lincoln, Victoria. *A Private Disgrace, Lizzie Borden by Daylight.* New York: G.P. Putnam's Sons, 1967.

Lipsitt, D.R. "Who Are the 'Worried Well'?" *General Hospital Psychiatry,* 4: 93-94, 1982.

MacKay, R.D. "Non-Organic Automatism — Some Recent Developments." *The Criminal Law Review,* 350-361, 1981.

MacLeod, Sheila. *The Art of Starvation.* New York: Schocken Books, 1982.

Mann, G.V. "Diet-Heart: End of an Era." *New England Journal of Medicine,* 297: 644, 1977.

Marker, R. "New Sources of Sapogenins." *Journal of American Chemical Society,* 69: 2242, 1947.

Marshall, J.L. *The Sports Doctors' Fitness Book for Women.* New York: Dell Publishing, 1981.

Martin, Clement G. *Low Blood Sugar: The Hidden Menace of Hypoglycemia.* New York: Arco Publishing Inc. 1969.

May, Rollo. *Power and Innocence.* New York: Delta Books, 1981.

McArthur, Janet W. "Common Menstrual Disorders in the Adolescent Girl." *Clinical Pediatrics,* 3, 11: 663, 1964.

McClintock, Martha K. "Menstrual Synchrony and Suppression." *Nature,* 229, 244: 5282, 1971.

McCullers, Carson. *The Member of the Wedding.* New York: Bantam Books, 1950.

McEwen, B.S. "Binding and Metabolism of Sex Steroids by the Hypothalamic-Pituitary Unit: Physiological Implications." *Annual Review of Physiology,* 42: 97, 1980.

McKinlay, Sonja M. and Jefferys, Margot. "The Menopausal Syndrome." *British Journal of Preventive and Social Medicine,* 28, 2: 108, 1974.

Mead, Margaret. *Male and Female.* New York: Dell Publishing Company, 1970.

Mead, Margaret. *Sex and Temperament.* New York: William Morrow & Company, 1935.

Meldrum, D.R. "Weighing Benefits and Risks of Hormone Therapy in the Menopause." *Contemporary OB/GYN,* 17: 157, 1981.

Mindell, E. *Vitamin Bible*. New York: Warner Books, 1979.

Mishell, D.R. "Noncontraceptive Health Benefits of Oral Steroidal Contraceptives." *American Journal of Obstetrics and Gynecology*, 809-816, March 1982.

Mitchell, Juliet. *Psychoanalysis and Feminism*. New York: Pantheon Books, 1974.

Moghissi, Kamran J. et al. "A Composite Picture of the Menstrual Cycle." *American Journal of Obstetrics and Gynecology*, 114, 3: 405-418, October 1, 1972.

Montagu, Ashley. *The Natural Superiority of Women*. New York: Collier Books, 1952.

Moore, Brian. *I Am Mary Dunne*. New York: The Viking Press, 1966.

Moos, Rudolph H. "Typology of Menstrual Cycle Symptoms." *American Journal of Obstetrics and Gynecology*, 103, 3: 390-402, February 1, 1968.

Morton, Joseph H. "Premenstrual Tension." *American Journal of Obstetrics and Gynecology*, 60: 343-352, 1950.

Morton, Joseph H. et al. "A Clinical Study of Premenstrual Tension." *American Journal of Obstetrics and Gynecology*, 65: 1182-1191, 1953.

Morton, Joseph H. ed. "Symposium on Premenstrual Tension." *International Record of Medicine*, 166, 11, November 1953.

Mukherjee. "Premenstrual Tension: A Critical Study of the Syndrome." *Journal of the Indian Medical Association*, 1954.

Naftolin, Frederick and Tolis, George. "Neuroendocrine Regulation of the Menstrual Cycle." *Clinical Obstetrics and Gynecology*, 21, 1: 17-29, March 1978.

Nathanson, Constance. "Illness and the Feminine Role: A Theoretical Review." *Social Science and Medicine*, 9: 57-62, 1975.

Nathanson, Constance. "Sex, Illness and Medical Care: A Review of Data, Theory and Method." *Social Science and Medicine*, 11: 13-25, 1977.

Nillius, S.J. and Johansson, E.D. "Plasma Levels of Progesterone After Vaginal, Rectal or Intramuscular Administration of Progesterone." *American Journal of Obstetrics and Gynecology,* 110: 470-477, June 1971.

O'Connor, J.F. et al. "Behavioral Rhythms Related to the Menstrual Cycle." *International Institue for the Study of Human Reproduction.* New York, 1973.

Okey, Ruth and Robb, Elda I. "Studies of the Metabolism of Women. Variations in the Fasting Blood Sugar Level and in Sugar Tolerance in Relation to the Menstrual Cycle." *Journal of Biological Chemistry,* 65: 165-189, 1925.

Oleck, Howard L. "Legal Aspects of Premenstrual Tension." *International Record of Medicine,* 166: 492-501, November 1953.

Ortzen, Len. *Imperial Venus.* New York: Stein and Day, 1974.

Parker, A. Seymour. "The Premenstrual Tension Syndrome." *Medical Clinics of North America,* 44: 339-347, November 7, 1960.

Parlee, Mary Brown. "The Premenstrual Syndrome." *Psychological Bulletin,* 80, 6: 454-465, 1973.

Pavese, Cesare. *This Business of Living,* translated by A.E. Murch. London and Toronto, 1961.

Pelletier, K.R. *Holistic Medicine: From Stress to Optimum Health.* New York: Dell Publishing, 1979.

Permutt, M.A. "Postprandial Hypoglycemia." *Diabetes,* 22: 719, 1976.

Pitt, Bruce. "Maternity Blues." *British Journal of Psychiatry,* 122: 431-433, 1973.

Plath, Sylvia. *The Bell Jar.* New York: Bantam Books, 1972.

Plath, Sylvia. *The Collected Poems.* New York: Harper and Row Publishers, 1981.

Plath, Sylvia. *The Journals of Sylvia Plath.* New York: Dial Press, 1982.

Pliny, *Natural History,* Book 7, translated by H. Rackham. Cambridge, Mass.: Harvard University Press, 1961.

Ploss, Hermann Heinrich et al. *Woman: An Historical Gynaecological and Anthropological Compendium.* St. Louis: Mosby, 1936.

Plowden, Alison. *Marriage With My Kingdom.* New York: Stein and Day, 1977.

Pratt, J.P. and Thomas, W.L. "The Endocrine Treatment of Menopausal Phenomena." *Journal of the American Medical Association,* 65, 1937.

Price, Trevor R.P. "Temporal Lobe Epilepsy as a Premenstrual Behavioral Syndrome." *Biological Psychiatry,* 15, 6: 957-963, 1980.

Putnam-Jacobi, Mary. *The Question of Rest for Women during Menstruation.* New York, 1877.

Raj, S., et al. "Clincial Aspects of the Polycystic Ovary Syndrome." *Obstetrics and Gynecology,* 49: 552, 1977.

Ramey, Estelle. "Men's Cycles (They Have Them Too, You Know)." *Ms.,* 8-14, Spring 1972.

Randall, Ruth Painter. *Mary Lincoln — Biography of a Marriage.* Boston: Little Brown and Company, 1953.

Rebeta-Burditt, Joyce. *The Cracker Factory.* New York: Bantam Books, 1978.

Rees, Linford. "The Premenstrual Tension Syndrome and Its Treatment." *British Medical Journal,* 1014-1016, May 9, 1953.

Reid, Robert L. and Yen, S.S.C. "Premenstrual Syndrome." *American Journal of Obstetrics and Gynecology,* 139: 85-104, 1981.

Reid, Robert L., "Premenstrual Syndrome: A Therapeutic Enigma." *Drug Therapy,* 33-43, April 1982.

Robbins, Fred P. "Psychosomatic Aspects of Dysmenorrhea." *American Journal of Obstetrics and Gynecology,* 66: 808-815, 1953.

Romney, S.L. et al. eds. *Gynecology and Obstetrics.* New York: McGraw-Hill Inc., 1981.

Rosenwaks, Z. "New Approach to Dysmenorrhea." *Drug Therapy*, 47-53, April 1982.

Rothchild, J. and Rappaport, R.S. "The Thermogenic Effect of Progesterone and Its Relation to Thyroid Function." *Endocrinology*, 50: 580, 1952.

Ryan, A.J. and Allman, F.L. *Sports Medicine*. New York: Academic Press, 1974.

Salhanick, H.A. et al. eds. *Metabolic Effects of Gonadal Hormones and Contraceptive Steroids*. New York: Plenum Press, 1969.

Sammour, Mohamed B. et al. "Progesterone Therapy in Pre-Eclamptic Toxaemia," *Acta Obstetrica Gynecologica Scandinavica*, 54: 195-202, 1975.

Sampson, Gwyneth A. "Premenstrual Syndrome: A Double-Blind Controlled Trial of Progesterone and Placebo." *British Journal of Psychiatry*, 135: 209-215, 1979.

Sampson, Gwyneth A. "An Appraisal of the Role of Progesterone in the Therapy of Premenstrual Syndrome," in van Keep, P.A., ed., *The Premenstrual Syndrome*. Lancaster, England: MTP Press Ltd., Falcon House International Medical Publishers, 51-69, 1981.

Samuels, Alec. "Psychiatric Evidence." *The Criminal Law Review*, 762-770, 1981.

Sanders, Lawrence. *The Third Deadly Sin*. New York: Berkley Books, 1982.

Sandmaier, Marian. *The Invisible Alcoholics*. New York: McGraw-Hill Inc., 1981.

Scarf, Maggie. *Unfinished Business*. New York: Ballantine Books, 1981.

Schwab, John J. "Psychiatric Illness in Medical Patients: Why It Goes Undiagnosed." *Psychosomatics*, 23, 3: 225-229, March 1982.

Scida, Joan and Vannicella, Marsha. "Sex-Role Conflict and Women's Drinking." *Journal of Studies on Alcohol*, 40, 1: 25-44, 1979.

Seelig, Mildred S. "The Requirement of Magnesium by the Normal Adult." *American Journal of Clinical Nutrition*, 14: 342-390, June 1979.

Selye, Hans. *The Physiology and Pathology of Exposure to Stress*. Montreal, Canada: Acta Inc., 1950.

Selye, Hans. *The Stress of Life*. New York: McGraw-Hill Inc., 1956.

Shader, Richard I. and Ohly, Jane I. "Premenstrual Tension, Femininity and Sexual Drive." *Medical Aspects of Human Sexuality*, April 1970.

Shainess, Natalie. "Psychiatric Evaluation of Premenstrual Tension." *New York State Journal of Medicine*, 3573-3579, November 15, 1962.

Shakespeare, William. *The Tragedy of Hamlet*, Prince of Denmark. New York: Washington Square Press, 1958.

Shangold, Mona. "The Relationship Between Long-Distance Running, Plasma Progesterone, and Luteal Phase Length." *Fertility and Sterility*, 31, 130: 607-608, 1979.

Sheehy, Gail. *Passages*. New York: E.P. Dutton Inc., 1974.

Siiteri, Pentti K. "Progesterone and Maintenance of Pregnancy: Is Progesterone Nature's Immunosuppressant?" *Annals of the New York Academy of Science*, 286: 434-445, March 1979.

Silber, Sherman J. *The Male*. New York: Charles Scribner's and Sons, 1981.

Smith, Bushnell and Prockop, Darwin. "Central-Nervous System Effects of Ingestion of L-Tryptophan by Normal Subjects." *New England Journal of Medicine*, 1338-1342, December 27, 1962.

Smith, O.W. and Smith, G. van S. "Menstrual Toxin," in *Menstruation and Its Disorders*, E.T. Engle ed. Springfield, Ill.: Charles C Thomas Publisher, 1950.

Smith, Stuart L. and Sauder, Cynthia. "Food Cravings, Depression, and Premenstrual Problems." *Psychosomatic Medicine*, XXXI, 4: 281-287, 1969.

Sommer, Barbara. "Menstrual Cycle Changes and Intellectual Performance." *Psychosomatic Medicine,* 35, 6: 515-534, Nov-Dec 1973.

Sontag, Susan. *Illness as Metaphor.* New York: Farrar, Straus and Giroux, 1977.

Soranus. *Gynecology,* translated by Owsei Temkin. Baltimore: Johns Hopkins University Press, 1956.

Southam, Anna L. and Gonzaga, Florante P. "Systemic Changes During the Menstrual Cycle." *American Journal of Obstetrics and Gynecology,* 91, 1: 142-165, January 1, 1965.

Speidel, J.J. et al. "Symposium on Oral Contraceptives." *The Johns Hopkins Medical Journal,* 150: 161-180, May 1982.

Speroff, Leon and Vande Wiele, Raymond. "Regulation of the Human Menstrual Cycle." *American Journal of Obstetrics and Gynecology,* 109, 2: 232-247, January 15, 1971.

Speroff, L. et al. *Clinical Gynecologic Endocrinology and Infertility.* Baltimore: Williams and Wilkins Company, 1978.

Spodick, D.H. "The Randomized Controlled Clinical Trials." *The American Journal of Medicine,* 73: 420-425, 1982.

Stadel, Bruce V. "Oral Contraceptives and Cardiovascular Disease." *New England Journal of Medicine,* 612-677. September 10, 1981.

Stassinopoulos, Arianna. *Maria Callas.* New York: Ballantine Books, 1982.

Steiner, Franz. *Taboo.* Baltimore: Penguin Books, 1956.

Steiner, Meir and Carroll, Bernard J. "The Psychology of Premenstrual Dysphoria: Review of Theories and Treatments." *Psychoneuroendocrinology,* 2: 321-335, 1977.

Stengel, Erwin. *Suicide and Attempted Suicide,* revised edition. Harmondsworth, 1969.

Stephens, William N. *A Cross-cultural Study of Menstrual Taboos.* Provincetown, Mass: Genetic Psych. Monographs, 1961.

Stoeckle, John D. "The Quantity and Significance of Psychological Distress in Medical Patients." *Journal of Chronic Diseases,* 17: 959-970, 1964.

Strouse, Jean. *Alice James.* New York: Bantam Books, 1982.

Suarez-Morias, Edward L. "The Psychophysiologic Syndrome of Premenstrual Tension with Emphasis on the Psychiatric Aspect." *International Record of Medicine,* 166,11: 475-486, November 1953.

Szpmtagh, F.E., *Mechanism of Action of Oral Progestogens.* Budapest: Akademai Kiado, 1970.

Tager, Benjamin N. and Kost, Shelton. "Personality Changes in Endocrine Disorders." *Journal of Clinical Endocrinology and Metabolism,* 239-242, 1943.

Tannahill, Reay. *Sex in History.* New York: Scarborough Books, 1982.

Terkel, Studs. *Working.* New York: Avon Books, 1975.

Thorne, G.W. "Cyclical Edema." *American Journal of Medicine,* 23: 507, 1957.

Tingsten, Herbert. *Victoria and the Victorians.* New York: Delacorte Press, 1972.

Timonen, Sakari and Procope, Berndt-Johan. "Premenstrual Syndrome and Physical Exercise." *Acta Obstetrica Gynecologica Scandinavica,* 50: 331-337, 1971.

Tolstoy, Leo. *Anna Karenina.* New York: Signet Classics, 1961.

Udry, J.R. and Morris, N. "Distribution of Coitus in the Menstrual Cycle." *Nature,* 220: 593, November 1968.

Van Keep, P.A. and Utian, W.H. *The Premenstrual Syndrome.* Lancaster, England: MTP Press Limited, 1981.

Vander, Arthur J. et al. *Human Physiology.* New York: McGraw-Hill Inc., 1970.

Verbrugge, Lois M. "Females and Illness: Recent Trends in Sex Differences in the United States." *Journal of Health and Social Behavior,* 17: 387-403, 1976.

Verbrugge, Lois M. ''Sex Differences in Morbidity and Mortality in the United States.'' *Social Biology,* 23: 275-296, 1977.

Verbrugge, Lois M. ''Sex and Gender in Health and Medicine.'' *Social Science and Medicine,* 12: 329-333, 1978.

Verbrugge, Lois M. ''Social Roles and Health Status Among Women: The Significance of Employment.'' *Social Science and Medicine,* 14A: 463-471, 1980.

Wallach, Aleta and Rubin, Larry. ''The Premenstrual Syndrome and Criminal Responsibility.'' *UCLA Law Review,* 19: 210-312, 1971.

Webster, Hutton. *Taboo - A Sociological Study.* Stanford, Calif.: Stanford University Press, 1942.

Weideger, Paula. *Menstruation and Menopause.* New York: Alfred A. Knopf, 1976.

Welner, Amos. ''Childbirth-Related Psychiatric Illness.'' *Comprehensive Psychiatry,* 23, 2: 143-154, March/April 1982.

Wentz, Anne Colston. ''Assessment of Estrogen and Progestin Therapy in Gynecology and Obstetrics.'' *Clinical Obstetrics and Gynecology,* 20, 2: 461-480, June 1977.

Wetzel, Richard D. et al. ''Premenstrual Symptoms in Self-Referrals to a Suicide Prevention Service.'' *British Journal of Psychiatry,* 119: 525-526, 1971.

Wetzel, Richard D. and McClure, J.N., Jr. ''Suicide and the Menstrual Cycle.'' *Comprehensive Psychiatry,* 13, 4: 369, 1972.

Whalen, Richard E. ed. *Hormones and Behavior.* Princeton, N.J.: D. Van Nostrand Company, 1967.

Whitehead, M.I. et al. ''Absorption and Metabolism of Oral Progesterone.'' *British Medical Journal,* 1: 825, 1980.

Whittlesey, Marietta. *Killer Salt.* New York: Avon Books, 1978.

Williams, E.Y. and L.R. Weekes. ''Premenstrual Tension Associated with Psychotic Episodes.'' *Journal of Nervous and Mental Disease,* 116: 321-329, 1952.

Williams, R.H. *Textbook of Endocrinology*. Philadelphia: W.B. Saunders Company, 1981.

Wise, Penny W. *No More Menstrual Cramps and Other Good News*. New York: Penguin Books, 1981.

Witzmann, R.F. *Steroids*. New York: Van Nostrand Reinhold, 1977.

Yager, J. and Young, R.T. "Non-hypoglycemia is an Epidemic Condition." *New England Journal of Medicine*, 291: 907, 1974.

Yen, S.S.C. et al. "Hormonal Relationships During the Menstrual Cycle." *Journal of the American Medical Association*, 211, 9: 1513-1517, March 2, 1970.

Index

P

PMS Action 287, 288
PMS Program Inc. 288
panic attacks 4, 116, 117
paranoia 108
Parker, Dorothy 138
Pavese, Cesare 132
pelvic inflammatory disease 13, 145
penis envy 18, 19, 47
periodic paralysis 107
periodic psychosis of puberty 164
Phil Donahue Show, The 129, 278
Pill, the. See Oral Contraceptives
pituitary gland 3, 6-8, 235
placenta 9
Plath, Sylvia 257, 265, 267, 268
Pliny the Elder 17
post-menopausal women 8
postpartum depression 11, 151-156
post-traumatic stress disorder 276
potassium 209
pregnancy 10, 11, 147-149
    and euphoria 147
    and toxemia 148
    multiple births 149
    multiple pregnancies 149
    see also
        abortion
        miscarriages
Premarin 40
premenstrual syndrome
    and adolescence 163-168
    and child abuse 4, 128-130
    and children 44, 63, 64, 92-101
    and divorce 87-90
    and the family 22, 44, 63-65, 77-101
    and husbands 22, 44, 63, 65, 126-128
    and menopause 179-182
    and suicide attempts 4, 131-138
    and violence 119-130
    as a legal defense 269-282
    genetic disposition to 67-74
    onset
        and amenorrhea 10
        and breast feeding 11
        and hysterectomy 11, 157-159
        and oral contraceptives 10, 11, 15, 141-145

and pregnancy 10, 11, 147-149
and puberty 10
and tubal ligation 11, 157-159
symptoms
    acne 3
    alcohol abuse 59-66
    anger 4
    anorexia nervosa 56, 57
    anxiety attacks 4, 33, 116, 117
    arthritis 22
    asthma 4
    binge eating 53, 54
    boils 4
    breast swelling 3, 21
    bulimia 56, 57
    conjunctivitis 22
    constipation 4
    crying spells 44, 45
    depression 3, 22, 43-49, 52, 55, 56
    dizziness 4
    drug abuse 59, 62, 66, 167, 168
    epilepsy 4, 22
    fatigue 22
    food cravings 3, 53-55
    fluid retention 3, 22, 24, 33
    gall bladder attacks 22
    headaches 3, 243
        migraine 4, 29-33
        muscle-contraction 33
        tension 33
    herpes 4, 22
    hives 4
    hypoglycemia 23, 24, 33, 201-205
    insomnia 159
    irritability 22, 33, 44
    jaundice 22
    mood swings 44, 45, 46
    paranoia 108
    periodic paralysis 107
    periodic psychosis of puberty 164
    postpartum depression 24, 151-156
    rhinitis 4
    sties 4
    thirst 3
    urethritis 4
    uveitis 4
    weight gain 3

NEW EYE-OPENING INSIGHTS FOR YOU ON LOVE AND MEN

__FINDING LOVE___ 0-515-09796-9/$3.95
Sally Jessy Raphael
"Gutsy, insightful and creative...A clear and concise book about what really counts in a relationship." –PHIL DONAHUE

__MEN WHO CAN'T LOVE___ 0-425-11170-9/$4.50
Steven Carter and Julia Sokol
This New York Times bestseller tells you how to recognize a commitment-phobic man before he breaks your heart.

__WHY MEN ARE THE WAY___ 0-425-11094-X/$4.95
THEY ARE
Warren Farrell, Ph.D.
A book for men and women explaining what men really feel and want. "The most important book ever written about love, sex, and intimacy."
–NEW YORK POST

__SUCCESSFUL WOMEN,___ 0-515-09653-9/$3.95
ANGRY MEN
Bebe Moore Campbell
Practical advice for the career woman whose spouse resents her success. "Thoughtful advice on ways couples can reduce stress." –Kirkus